WEANING
and First Foods

NICOLA GRAIMES

hamlyn

An Hachette UK company
www.hachette.co.uk

First published in Great Britain in 2009 by
Carroll & Brown Publishers Limited

This second edition published in 2015 by Hamlyn,
a division of Octopus Publishing Group Ltd
Endeavour House, 189 Shaftesbury Avenue
London WC2H 8JY
www.octopusbooksusa.com

Distributed in the US by
Hachette Book Group
1290 Avenue of the Americas
4th and 5th Floors
New York, NY 10020

Distributed in Canada by
Canadian Manda Group
664 Annette St.
Toronto, Ontario, Canada M6S 2C8

ISBN 978-0-600-63167-5

Printed and bound in China

10 9 8 7 6 5 4 3 2 1
-

All reasonable care has been taken in the preparation of this
book but the information it contains is not intended to take
the place of treatment by a qualified medical practitioner.

The U.S. Department of Agriculture advises that eggs should
not be consumed raw. This book contains dishes made with
raw or lightly cooked eggs. It is prudent for more vulnerable
people, such as pregnant and nursing mothers, people with
weakened immune systems, the elderly, babies, and young
children, to avoid uncooked or lightly cooked dishes made with
eggs. Once prepared these dishes should be kept refrigerated
and used promptly.
This book includes dishes made with nuts and nut derivatives. It
is advisable for customers with known allergic reactions to nuts
and nut derivatives and those who may be potentially
vulnerable to these allergies, such as pregnant and nursing
mothers, people with weakened immune systems, the elderly,
babies, and children, to avoid dishes made with nuts and nut
oils. It is also prudent to check the labe--ls of prepared
ingredients for the possible inclusion of nut derivatives.

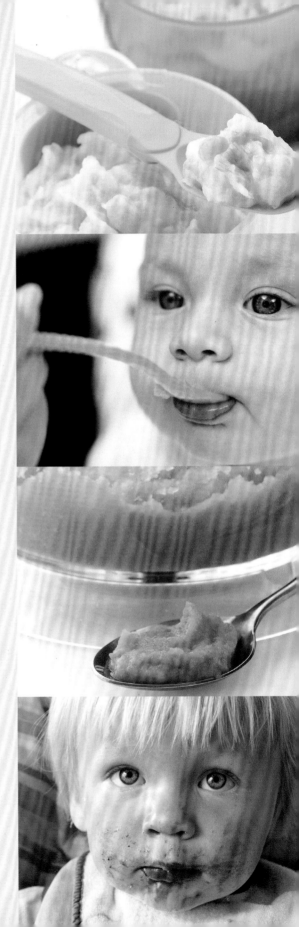

CONTENTS

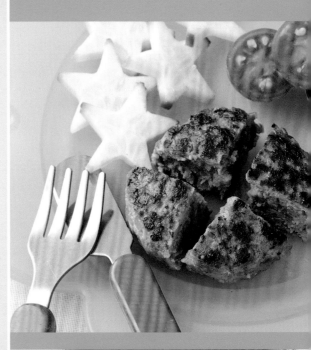

Many parents feel slightly daunted by the prospect of weaning their baby, and I can recall feeling exactly the same with my daughter. I had got to grips with breastfeeding, but the next stage of actually introducing solid food to her diet was somewhat scary—a journey into the unknown. The combination of a desire to do the best for her and the various pieces of advice from well-meaning friends and family conspired to add to my uncertainty. My nervousness was unnecessary, because weaning wasn't as difficult as I had predicted; however, I know my concerns were not out of the ordinary.

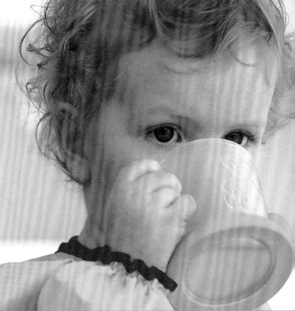

My aim in writing this book is to ease any concerns other parents may have and to give a practical and reassuring guide to feeding babies and toddlers. Welcome weaning as an exciting stage in your baby's life and a natural part of her development. Keep in mind that the principle of weaning (the process of replacing a baby's total dependence on milk with "solid" foods) is to gradually introduce her to a wide range of tastes and textures until she can eventually enjoy the same meals as the rest of the family. The emphasis is on proceeding gradually, so take it slowly and enjoy this new stage in your baby's development.

Be prepared for mess—and enjoy the ride.

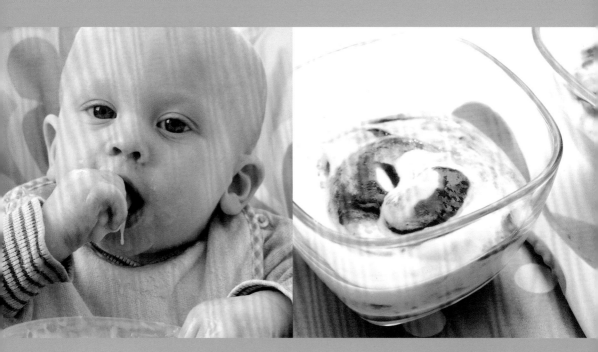
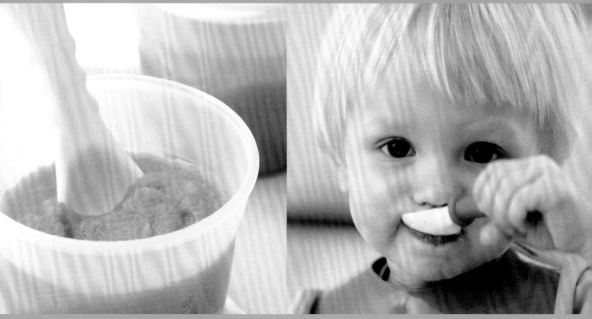

PREFACE

When to Start Weaning

Your baby should be ready to start solids at around six months. Until then, breast or formula milk meets all of your baby's dietary needs. There are no nutritional advantages to weaning before this age. And because your baby's immune system is not yet completely developed, there are good reasons not to start before the age of six months.

The American Academy of Pediatrics recommends that the majority of babies should start a mixed diet from the age of six months (26 weeks), by which time breast milk and formula do not meet all of their dietary needs. Before four months (17 weeks) a baby's digestive system is too immature to cope with anything more than breast milk or formula. It has been said that weaning too early may make a baby fat and increase the likelihood of allergies; waiting until your baby is six months old can reduce this risk, especially if there is a family history of weight problems and allergies.

However, the guidelines do not completely take into account the wide individual variations in developmental maturity (and appetite) between infants, and some are ready for solids slightly before they are six months old—talk to your child's healthcare provider if you are unsure. There are three key signs that indicate that your baby is physically ready to start solids: she can stay supported in a sitting position and hold her head steady; she can cooordinate her eyes and hands and pick food up and put it in her mouth by herself; and she can swallow. Signs that can be mistaken for a baby needing solid food, such as waking in the night after sleeping through, suddenly needing an extra milk feed, or chewing her fists, are normal behavior patterns for her age and don't necessarily mean that she is physically ready for solids.

Don't wait to start weaning much longer than six months, unless recommended by a healthcare provider, because after six months, babies need more nutrients than breast or formula milk provides, particularly of iron. Requirements for protein, thiamine, niacin, vitamins B_6 and B_{12}, magnesium, zinc, sodium, and chloride also increase between the ages of 6 and 12 months. Babies will only get this if they begin to have a varied diet with food from all the main food groups.

Babies who are born preterm need to be weaned according to their own individual needs and your healthcare provider or dietitian will be able to advise on the best time for your baby.

TO RECAP
- Weaning should be started when your baby is six months (24 weeks) old.
- From the age of six months, your baby's nutrient requirements increase, so she needs a diet that includes all the main food groups.
- If think your baby is ready for solid foods earlier, first discuss it with your healthcare provider or pediatrician.
- There are foods that must always be avoided before the age of six months.

STAGE 1: Introducing Solids

Weaning is all about getting your baby used to moving food around her mouth that is not liquid. While most foods are suitable for your baby from six months (see page 9 for the exceptions), it's advisable to start gradually, especially if there is a family history of allergies or food intolerance. The first step is to simply familiarize your baby with taking food from a spoon; the food should be smooth, semi-iquid in consistency, with a bland flavor. Initially, the quantity eaten is largely immaterial. If your baby is allowed to feed herself, spoon feeding may develop later. Try sitting your baby at the table when you are eating so she gets used to the idea. She may want to try some of your food, too.

Choose a time of day when you are not feeling too rushed or your baby too tired to introduce solids; midday is often best. Keep in mind that eating is a new skill for your baby, so don't expect her to get it right from the start. She is using previously unused muscles, so don't be worried if food appears to be spat out at first—this is perfectly normal. Face-to-face interaction is important. Talk to your baby while you feed her; encourage and praise her.

Start gradually—offer some pureed fruit or vegetables (see page 8) on the tip of a plastic spoon or a clean finger. It may be a good idea to first give your baby a little milk to curb any hunger pangs, but as feeding becomes more established, start to offer food before milk. Don't expect your baby to eat more than 1–2 teaspoons at first—although she could eat more. The first solids should be regarded as a

did you know...
Until around six months of age, babies usually have a protective mechanism whereby the tongue pushes forward, but this then changes and babies begin to be able to take food to the back of the mouth. This explains why in the early stages of weaning, it appears that food is being "spat" or pushed out with the tongue.

supplement to your baby's milk feed, and you will find that her appetite will vary from one feed to another, so watching how much she is eating every day is not important at this stage. When she loses interest in the food, continue with milk.

For the first few weeks, offer the same food for around three days at a time to allow your baby to get used to new tastes. It is a good idea to keep a food diary to monitor likes and dislikes and gauge if there is any sign of an intolerance or allergy. Signs that your baby may have an allergy include a rash, diarrhea, bloated belly, or increased gas (see also page 17). Don't be surprised when your baby's stools change

? Is your baby ready

All babies are different and progress at their own pace, but the following signs may indicate that your baby is ready for weaning. Your baby:

✓ Can sit supported in a sitting position—for example, in a high chair.
✓ Shows an interest in your food.
✓ Makes chewing motions.
✓ Can close her mouth around a spoon.
✓ Holds her head up well.
✓ Can sit up with support.
✓ Can move her tongue back and forth, so she can swallow.
✓ Is teething.

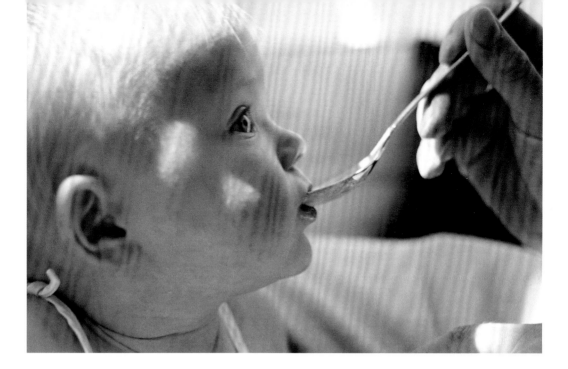

color and odor after starting solids. This is perfectly normal. Constipation also is not unusual at this stage. Baby rice cereal, for example, lacks fiber, and constipation may be due to dehydration or simply that the digestive

Face-to-face interaction is important. Talk to your baby through the feeding and try to be both encouraging and positive.

system is getting used to food. If your baby is constipated, try fruit and vegetables instead of rice, because they are richer in fiber, and offer cooled, boiled tap water in a cup (see page 11).

did you know...

Research from the Monell Chemical Senses Center in Philadelphia, Pennsylvania, suggests that young babies will probably be more successfully weaned on foods to which they have been exposed to in the womb, or through the traces that make it into breast milk—including broccoli and cabbage. These vegetables have naturally bitter flavors that children often dislike, but babies may be more open to the vegetables' tastes if they are already familiar with them.

Babies also are said to be particularly open to new tastes and textures between six to nine months. It has been suggested that parents try providing ingredients individually so infants can taste each one instead of mixing them together into a single mass.

FIRST FOODS

Start with mild-tasting, single-ingredient purees, for example, carrot, parsnip, apple, pear, or bananas. Wash or scrub them thoroughly, peel them, and remove any core and seeds before cooking. Or you could try dry baby rice cereal or home-cooked pureed white rice mixed with breast or formula milk. You can also add vegetables or fruit to the rice. At the early stage, foods should ideally be pureed to a semiliquid state—the texture of heavy cream (see page 15).

There is a selection of first food recipes on pages 42 to 45, followed by others suitable once weaning is becoming established. Keep in mind that the age recommendations given are a general guide; only give foods to your baby when you think she is ready to eat them.

FOODS TO AVOID

There are a number of seasonings and foodstuffs that should not be given to babies and toddlers (see page 20 for a more in-depth explanation).

Never give the following babies to under six months:

- Salt or hot spices
- Wheat and other grains containing gluten, such as barley and rye
- Eggs
- Unpasteurized cheese
- Meat, including liver, and poultry
- Honey and sugar
- Fish and shellfish
- Citrus fruit and juices
- Berries
- Nuts (including peanuts or peanut products) and seeds
- Follow-on formula milk and cow, goat, and sheep milk

Never give the following to babies between six months old and one year:

- Salt or hot spices
- Unpasteurized cheese
- Raw or soft-cooked eggs
- Honey and sugar
- Shellfish, such as shrimp or mussels
- Shark, swordfish, and marlin (these fish contain relatively high levels of mercury)
- Whole nuts—or any food containing nuts if there is a family history of food allergies
- Cow, sheep, and goat milk as a drink

MILK MATTERS

For the first year, breast or formula milk is a vital source of nutrients for your baby, but you may find that as she eats more solid foods, she naturally takes less milk. Yet, if she drinks too much milk, her appetite for solids could be affected and she may begin to lack sufficient nutrients in her diet. In the early stages of weaning, your baby should be still be having at least four bottles of formula or the equivalent number of breastfeeds a day.

KEEPING THINGS SAFE

Remember to wash your hands with soap before preparing meals and make sure the rest of the family does the same.

Be meticulous with hygiene and cleanliness and make sure all bowls and spoons are sterilized (or washed in the dishwasher) until weaning is established.

Avoid keeping any leftover food for future use or reheating food, because it could be a breeding ground for bacteria. Any leftover food should be thrown away.

Never leave your baby alone with food.

Give your baby her own baby-friendly utensils and always stay nearby when she is self-feeding. Take a first-aid class so you can help her if she chokes.

Always check the temperature of your baby's food before giving it to her. Be careful if you heat food in a microwave, because it can create hot spots.

If serving food from a jar, be sure that the seal is intact by listening for the popping sound when you open it. If the seal has been broken, the food must be thrown away. Spoon out a serving into a separate bowl and keep any remainder stored in the refrigerator for a maximum of 24 hours. If you buy prepared foods, they should be eaten by their expiration date.

Until she has enough teeth to chew, never give your baby grapes, raisins, cherry tomatoes, popcorn, olives, lumps of meat, cheese, or large pieces of raw vegetables.

GETTING EQUIPPED

There is no need to invest in large amounts of equipment, but the following are worth considering:

Bibs—you'll need plenty. There are many types to choose from, but the plastic-backed bibs prevent food and drinks from soaking through to clothes. Molded plastic bibs with a food-catching pocket are more suitable for slightly older babies who have started to feed themselves

Two or three shallow plastic feeding spoons

Two nonslip plastic bowls

Strainer or food grinder

Steamer—while not essential, steaming helps to retain water-soluble nutrients in fruit and vegetables

Feeder cup with two handles

Mini food processor, stand blender, or handheld immersion blender—again, not essential, but these make light work of pureeing and finely chopping meals

Cow (also sheep and goat) milk can be included in cooking from six months of age, but they are not recommended as a main drink until your baby is one year old, because they contain too much salt and protein and insufficient iron and other nutrients. A breastfed baby will take what she needs from the breast; it is not advisable to reduce breastfeeds, because there is no evidence that this will hinder her development. Give your baby soy-based formula milk only if prescribed by your pediatrician or healthcare provider. Continue to sterilize feeding bottles, because warm milk is a breeding ground for bacteria.

WATER
Before six months of age, fully breastfed babies should not require additional fluids, including

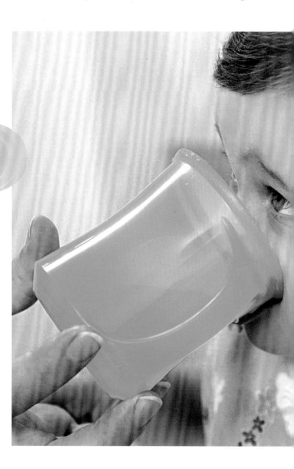

water, unless otherwise recommended. Bottle-fed babies may be given cooled, boiled tap water in hot weather, but this should be in addition to milk feeds.

When feeding is more established, your baby may need fluids other than milk. Cooled, boiled tap water is the preferred option; some mineral waters are too rich in minerals for babies and bottled water is not sterile. Avoid soft drinks and fruit juice; because they are high in sugar, they can damage teeth even before they appear. You can now drop the lunchtime milk feed. Start with a tablespoon of water in a cup with a lid and soft spout and increase the amount gradually as you increase the number of meals a day.

INTRODUCING A CUP

It is a good idea to get your baby used to drinking from a cup from about six months,

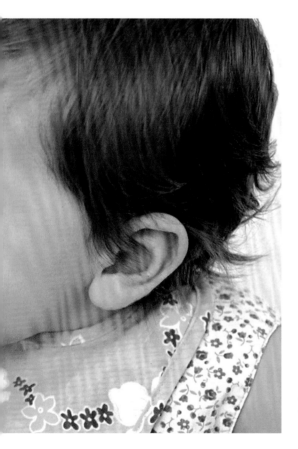

when you start feeding solids. If your baby has drunk only from a breast or bottle up until now, changing to a cup may be a challenge and some babies take time to accept the change. At first, to familiarize your baby with this new method of drinking, try offering some of her usual milk in a cup instead of water.

Because the object is for your baby to progress from sucking to drinking, open cups or free-flowing feeders are the recommended choices. Many parents, however, opt for a cup with a soft spout, a lid, and two handles, because it is easier for a young baby than a cup; they see it as a compromise between sucking and ordinary drinking that their baby will probably find more acceptable. It is important to keep in mind, however, that lidded and spouted cups encourage frequent sipping and have the potential to damage teeth, interfere with oral muscle development, and may even have a detrimental effect on speech.

Wash these cups in the dishwasher, because they can harbor bacteria. Be careful that you don't leave cups lying around. A baby can find a lost cup hours, or even days, after it was filled,

did you know...

Babies are born with a natural store of iron, and the mineral is also found in useful amounts in breast and formula milk. By six months of age, however, these iron reserves have largely been used up and even if your baby is breastfed or drinking iron-fortified milk, it is important to include foods rich in the mineral in your baby's diet. Good sources include red meat, liver, leafy green vegetables, beans and other legumes, eggs, fish, dried fruit (especially apricots), and fortified breakfast cereals.

A cup without a spout makes it easier for babies to drink without sipping, which has the potential to damage teeth.

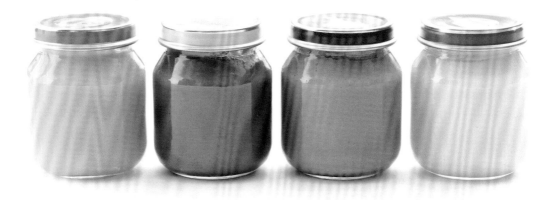

and she will be sucking on a drink that will probably be contaminated.

SUPPLEMENTS

The American Acadamy of Pediatrics encourages giving all babies (breast or bottle fed) an oral supplement of vitamin D, which is particularly important if your baby is dark-skinned or you live in an area with limited sunlight. If your baby is breastfeeding or drinking less than 33.8 ounces (just under 1 quart) of formula milk or follow-on milk, supplements may be recommended; talk to your healthcare provider.

FOCUS ON | additives

While the adverse health affects of artificial additives and preservatives on children have always been refuted, a study by the University of Southampton, England, has discovered that certain artificial food colors and preservatives, when combined, can adversely influence the behavior of children. Researchers believe the use of additives may help to explain the rise in attention deficit hyperactivity disorder (ADHD) and parents are advised to cut out some E-numbers and additives altogether.

The colors tested were tartrazine (E102), ponceau 4r (E124), quinoline yellow (E104), sunset yellow (E110), carmoisine (E122), and allura red (E129). It also looked at the preservative sodium benzoate (E211).

COMMERCIAL BABY FOODS

In an ideal world, we would all feed our babies nothing but home-prepared food, but a combination of homemade with the occasional jar of commercially made baby food is more realistic, manageable, and practical for most of us. There are now numerous organic baby food companies making both chilled and frozen meals, many of which are close in quality to home-prepared foods, albeit more costly. It is important when buying commercial baby foods to read the label carefully and to make sure that:

- The ingredients are suitable for your baby's age.
- There are no unwanted additives (see box, left); artificial sweeteners (aspartame, saccharine); sugars (dextrose, sucrose, glucose); salt; and thickeners, such as modified starch.
- The product has not passed its best before or expiration date.
- The seals are intact.

FOCUS ON | **baby-led weaning**

While current guidelines recommend that weaning begins with pureed food, Gill Rapley, a British health visitor who has specialized in young children's health for more than 25 years, thinks otherwise. She believes feeding babies pureed food is both unnecessary and unnatural and has pioneered what has become known as "Baby-Led Weaning," which centers on babies being in charge of what they eat and how much. The idea is that, instead of starting with purees, you present your child with a variety of healthy finger foods or meals made up of solid pieces of food that can be picked up— as long as your baby can sit in a high chair without being propped up.

Rapley believes that spoon-feeding pureed food to children could cause health problems later in life and blames the multimillion dollar baby food industry for convincing parents that they need to first wean their babies on pureed food . However, offering babies pureed food once they can chew is not only unnecessary, says Rapley, but also could delay chewing skills. In addition, allowing a child to eat as much or as little as she chooses could prevent her from becoming constipated. Constipation can trouble many babies not long after solids are introduced; it's not certain why, but it may be due to spoon-fed babies being given more food than they need or with which they can cope.

Ideally, says Rapley, a baby should be fed exclusively breast milk or formula until six months, and then weaned immediately onto finger food, because she has found that babies are capable of chewing at this age. They don't need teeth to chew; their gums work well. Ideally, food should be cut into

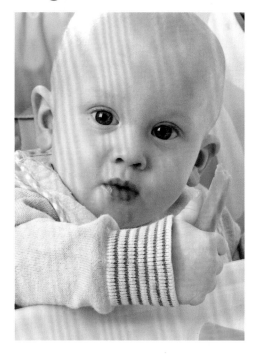

baby fist-size sticks, because this shape provides a baby with a handle ideal for grasping the food. Babies will chew the part sticking out of their fists and drop the rest later on.

Rapley believes that babies allowed to feed themselves tend to become less picky, develop better hand control more quickly, and appear to avoid foods to which they were later found to be intolerant. Another advantage is that babies can eat what you're eating and there is no need for pureeing.

Many pediatricians are interested in her findings, but some feel that purees could help some babies make the transition between liquid and solid foods more easily. The general feeling is that all babies are different and the suggestion that one size fits all is inappropriate.

STAGE 2: Increasing The Menu

If your baby is happy eating one "meal" a day (probably a few tablespoons), then now is the time to increase the number to two and eventually three in the next few weeks or so. Start adding different foods to familiarize your baby with new tastes and flavor combinations and you will definitely reap the benefits, because studies have found that children who have been exposed to a variety of foods from an early age are less likely to be fussy eaters later on in life. Researchers have found that between the ages of six to nine months, children are more receptive to new tastes and textures and their experiences during this period are thought to define their palate in later life.

Do remember that all babies are different—some take to weaning readily, happy to accept new foods, while others take longer. Don't panic or rush things; most important, try to make sure mealtimes are as happy and relaxed as possible and not occasions for power games.

COOKING FOR YOUR BABY

It is widely believed that good eating habits are formed early, so it's important at this stage to introduce a wider range of fresh foods, including a greater choice of fruit and vegetables, carbohydrates, and proteins.

Carbohydrates include rice, pasta, noodles, potatoes, bread, grains, and oats and other cereals, while fish, meat, poultry, regular dairy products, well-cooked eggs, legumes (beans and lentils), tofu, and meat alternatives are proteins. (For more information, see page 19.)

You'll probably find many of your meals, such as thick soups, pasta in tomato sauce, or vegetables in cheese sauce are suitable for your baby, but avoid adding any seasoning, such as salt and hot spices, at this stage. Be aware that processed foods may contain sugar, salt, and preservatives, as well as milk in various forms, such as whey powder.

There are no hard or fast rules on how much your baby should be eating now, but around one to four tablespoons per meal is the general guideline. Try to respond to your baby's appetite; if he is still hungry, then you can give him a little more, but don't force him to eat if he has eaten only a small amount, because this is bound to backfire. At this stage, move on from runny purees to more chunky purees and even mashed or ground foods. (Alternatively, see the information on Baby-Led Weaning, page 13.) If your baby spits out any lumps at first, which is not unusual, don't rush this change but gradually increase the texture of his food, making it lumpier and slightly more of a challenge to eat.

Some babies prefer the individual ingredients in their meals to be kept separate, so that they

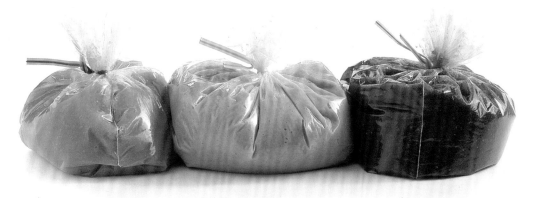

FOCUS ON | **preparing food**

The texture of your baby's food should keep pace with his progress. Start by pureeing food to an almost liquid consistency, then gradually process for a shorter time in the blender so the food is lumpier. From here, you can mash, grind, or finely chop the ingredients.

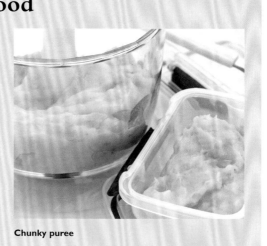

Chunky puree

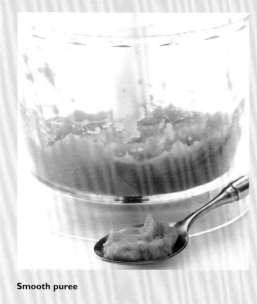

Smooth puree

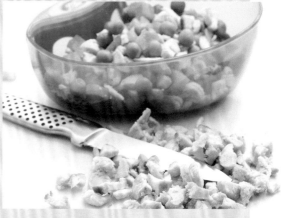

Chopped chicken

can log and identify each taste and texture. This makes sense in many ways but obviously the food has to be presented in a form with which your baby can cope.

In many ways, homemade meals are just as convenient and are certainly cheaper than commercially made alternatives, and many of your meals will now be suitable for your baby.

Storing and reheating food

It is a good idea to prepare baby meals in bulk and freeze them. If storing meals for later use, cool food as quickly as possible (ideally within 1–2 hours) then place in the refrigerator. Food can be divided into single portions at this stage, then refrigerated for up to two days.

If freezing, wrap single portions in freezer-safe plastic wrap or place in ice cube trays. Make sure you label and date the food packages. When you want to use them, remove from the plastic wrap or ice cube tray. The safest way to defrost food is to store frozen food in the refrigerator overnight or use the defrost setting on a microwave or oven.

Reheat foods thoroughly when defrosted. Once piping hot, stir well to remove any hot spots and let cool until it is the right temperature for your baby to eat. If anything is left over, discard it immediately; do not reheat, refreeze, or reuse under any circumstances (due to the risk of food poisoning).

ORGANIC FOODS

While you may have to pay a little more for organic foods, the benefits are numerous. There is good evidence to suggest a connection between pesticide residues and allergies and hyperactivity in children.

Fresh organic produce tends to taste better because it is not intensively grown to absorb excess water and is generally grown in better-quality soil and left to ripen for longer. Studies have shown that the lower levels of water in fresh organic produce means that it has higher concentrations of nutrients.

FINGER FOODS

You will probably find your baby loves finger foods. Not only do finger foods help to soothe sore gums and make great snacks, but they also encourage independence through self-feeding. Your baby is probably starting to cut a few teeth now and finger foods will allow him to practice chewing and keep him occupied when you are preparing his food or the family meal.

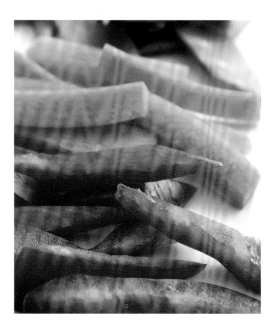

Make sure fingers foods are not too small or awkward to hold. Ideally, food should be cut into baby fist-size sticks, which makes it easy for a baby to grasp and eat. Never leave your baby alone when he is feeding so you can be sure he doesn't choke. Remember to remove any core, skin, or seeds from fruit. Try to avoid giving sweet cookies or rusks because these will encourage a sweet tooth and lead to weight increase and tooth decay.

Choose from
- Steamed vegetables, such as carrot sticks, snow peas, green beans, baby corn, or strips of red bell pepper, chunks of sweet potato, broccoli, and asparagus.
- Fruit, such as peeled wedges of apple or pear, and pieces of banana, mango, melon, or peach.
- Large cooked pasta shapes.
- Bread sticks, rice cakes, or fingers of bread, toas,t or pita bread.

MILK AND DRINKS

Breast milk, formula milk, or follow-on milk continue to be the main source of nutrients, including iron, for your baby: 2 to 2½ cups (16 to 20 ounces) daily is recommended. However, if you haven't done so already and feeding is established, you now can drop the lunchtime milk feed and provide a feeder cup of cooled boiled tap water (you may find that he naturally becomes less interested in the bottle and happy to take a cup). At other mealtimes, offer milk after his meal to prevent him from becoming too full or preoccupied with the bottle before he has eaten solid foods.

Do not give your baby cow, sheep, or goat milk as a drink, but it can now be used in cooking, such as in sauces or desserts.

Steam vegetables until your baby has cut a few teeth and is familiar with finger foods.

FOCUS ON | **allergies**

Statistics show that the number of children with food intolerances and allergies is on the rise, although the number of infants with life-threatening allergies remains relatively small. The prevalence of nut allergy, however, has tripled in the last 20 years and affects about three million people in the United States.

Many food intolerances and allergies begin in early childhood and the most common allergens are nuts (particularly peanuts), seeds, cow milk, wheat, gluten, eggs, berries, citrus fruit, tomatoes, sugar, and seafood. With a food intolerance, the body struggles to digest a particular food. A food intolerance can develop over a period of time—even into adulthood. With a food allergy, however, the immune system has an immediate adverse reaction to a particular food or trigger. An allergic reaction is potentially serious, but it is also far more rare than a food intolerance. Intolerances can be difficult to detect because symptoms are wide ranging, including colic, upset stomach, rashes, and hyperactivity to asthma and eczema. Anaphylactic shock, a severe life-threatening allergic reaction, can begin with minor symptoms, such as generalized rash and flushed appearance, but it can quickly develop into swelling of the face and mouth, difficulty swallowing, and severe breathing difficulties. Anaphylaxis needs urgent medical attention; so call an ambulance if you notice any of the symptoms.

It is recommended that common allergenic foods are introduced into the diet gradually and one at a time, which allows you to monitor for any adverse reaction.

Children are more susceptible than adults to food intolerance, because they have immature digestive and immune systems. Intolerances and allergies both tend to run in families. Babies who face the highest risk of nut allergy, for example, are those with immediate family members who have a nut allergy or other allergic conditions such as asthma, eczema, and hay fever (known as "atopic" allergy). Children who have one parent with an allergy carry a 30 percent risk of developing a condition, but having two such parents pushes the risk up to 70 percent. It is recommended that babies at risk should not be given nuts and nut-related products until the age of three, and that parents try to be vigilant when reading food labels because just a small amount of nuts in a product can cause a severe reaction.

There is no need to avoid nuts or nut products if there are no cases of intolerances or allergies within the family, particularly because they are be nutritious. However, make sure they are ground, finely chopped, or crushed if giving them to young children, because they are a choking risk.

If there is a history of food allergies in the family or, indeed, hay fever, eczema, and asthma, consult your pediatrician or health-care profession about dietary restrictions.

Some allergies can be helped by eating a healthy, well-balanced diet that is low in sugar and additives. A diet containing plenty of different types of fruits and vegetables has been shown to play a preventive role for those have asthma, for example.

Note

All recipes containing nuts and seeds in the recipe section are highlighted.

STAGE 3: Three Meals A Day

If your baby is happy eating the meals you are giving her, from around the age of seven to nine months you can start to increase the number of solid feeds from two to three, if you have not done so already. Again, introduce new foods gradually, but try to make sure your baby is eating a range of foods to get a good balance of nutrients, particularly iron (see page 11). You will probably find that many family meals are suitable but avoid chili and hot spices and seasonings. Mashed, ground, or finely chopped foods will encourage your baby to chew.

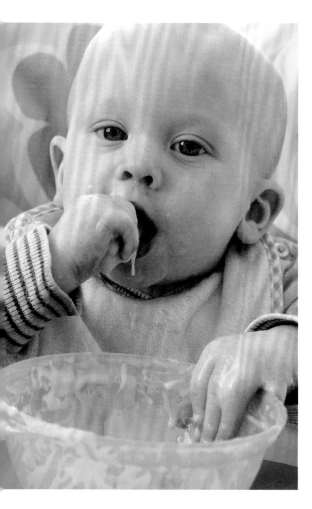

? Is your baby eating enough

At eight to nine months, your baby will start to enjoy three meals a day and will benefit from a varied diet based on the following:

✓ 3–4 servings a day of starchy carbohydrate foods, such as bread, pasta, rice, potatoes, and breakfast cereals.

✓ 2–3 servings a day of meat, fish, poultry, beans and other legumes, eggs, and dairy products.

✓ 3–4 servings a day of fruit and vegetables.

VEGETARIAN BABIES

With a little planning and attention, a vegetarian diet can provide all the nutrients a baby needs for growth and development. As with any diet, variety is the key. Make sure you provide protein from a variety of sources, including nuts (if there is no sign of an allergy within the family), seeds, eggs, dairy products, beans and other legumes—including lentils— and tofu, and combine with vitamin C-rich fruit and vegetables to aid iron absorption. A meat-free diet is naturally high in fiber, too much of which may result in an upset stomach, low energy intake, and interfere with the absorption of iron, zinc, and copper. For these reasons, avoid giving your baby, at least when especially young, large quantities of brown rice, whole-grain bread, or whole-wheat pasta. Try to make beans and other legumes a big part of your baby's diet; they are an important source of iron and also make a great base for many main dishes, such as soups and stews, and for dips. Make sure your baby is getting enough of the B vitamins, iron, and zinc (see page 21).

WHAT BABIES NEED

Babies grow a lot in the first year and have high energy requirements for their size. Aim to provide a good balance of especially fresh foods, but at this stage also think about how your baby's diet pans out over a week instead of on a daily basis: eating patterns can be erratic in infants, and you are still in the relatively early stages of weaning.

Carbohydrate/starchy foods (3–4 servings a day)

The following are an excellent source of energy, vitamins, minerals, and fiber (while a diet rich in fiber is perfect for adults, avoid giving too many high-fiber foods to babies, because they find them difficult to digest and can upset the digestive system):
• Sugar-free breakfast cereals and oats
• Pasta and noodles
• Rice
• Bread
• Potatoes

Protein foods (2–3 servings a day)

The following provide a good source of protein, essential for growth and repair in the body. Offer a combination of protein foods to get a good mix of essential amino acids:
• Fish
• Tofu
• Meat and poultry
• Meat alternatives
• Well-cooked eggs
• Regular cheese (grated or cubed)
• Beans and other legumes
• Yogurt or cottage cheese

Milk

Milk provides protein, vitamins, and minerals, particularly calcium for strong teeth and bones. Cow milk can be used in cooking from six months, but it should not given as a drink until your child is one year old, when regular milk can be introduced. Reduced-fat milk is suitable from two years, while skim milk is not recommended until five years of age, because it does not provide the energy a growing child requires.

Fruit and vegetables (3–4 or more servings a day)

Fresh, frozen, canned, and dried fruit and vegetables are an essential part of a baby's diet. They are ideal first foods and provide rich amounts of vitamins, especially vitamin C, minerals, and fiber. Foods that contain vitamin C (which is good for the immune system, hair, skin, and nails) should be included in meals, because they assist the absorption of iron. Try to provide your baby with a variety of fresh produce. The following are is short list of suitable foods:
• Peeled apple
• Banana
• Mango
• Apricots
• Peaches and nectarines
• Melon
• Strawberries
• Carrot
• Broccoli
• Green beans
• Peas
• Bell pepper
• Snow peas

FOODS TO AVOID IN EARLY CHILDHOOD

Whole nuts should never be given to children under five because of the risk of choking. However, all foods containing nuts should also be avoided if there is a history of food allergies within the immediate family (see page 17). Sliced, finely chopped nuts, or peanut butter are suitable from six months of age if there is no history of allergies.

Sugar is high in calories, nutritionally poor, and will ruin a child's appetite. It also leads to tooth decay and, if eaten in excess, may lead to obesity. Sugary foods often include a fair amount of fat—just think of doughnuts, cookies, and cakes.

Honey is a sugary food and causes similar health problems to those caused by sugar. It also occasionally contains a bacterium that has been known to cause infant botulism. For this reason, honey is not recommended for babies under one year (after this age the intestines are sufficiently mature to prevent the bacteria from growing).

Cow, sheep, or goat milks are not recommended as a drink for babies under one year, because they do not contain sufficient iron and other nutrients needed by infants.. However, from six months of age, these milks can be mixed into a baby's cooked dishes, such a cheese sauces, or poured over breakfast cereals.

Eggs should be cooked until both the white and yolk are solid. Raw or partly cooked eggs can be a source of salmonella, which can cause food poisoning, which can be particularly dangerous in vulnerable babies.

Salt can be harmful to a baby's immature kidneys if added to food—just 1 teaspoon of salt has 2,325mg of sodium. Up to seven months of age, babies should have less than 400mg of sodium a day; from 7 to 12 months, 400mg a day is the maximum recommended amount. Children between the ages of one and three years should have no more than 800mg of sodium a day. Naturally salty foods, such as bacon, cheese, broth, and yeast extract should be limited. Be aware that milk contains sodium, so babies are getting some sodium even when not eating many weaning foods.

Shellfish, such as shrimp and mussels, due to the slight risk of food poisoning.

Marlin, shark, and swordfish have been found to contain significant amounts of mercury, and it is recommended that you don't include these fish in a child's diet, because the mercury can affect the developing nervous system.

Foods high in saturated fat can be harmful to a child's health, increasing the risk of heart problems in later life as well as type 2 diabetes. Avoid giving too many fatty foods, such as butter, cheese, margarine, fatty meat and meat products, cookies, pastry, and cakes. Do not, however, avoid fats altogether; they are needed for nerve development. Instead, make sure your baby eats foods rich in omega-3 and omega-6 fatty acids, such as oily fish and vegetable oils.

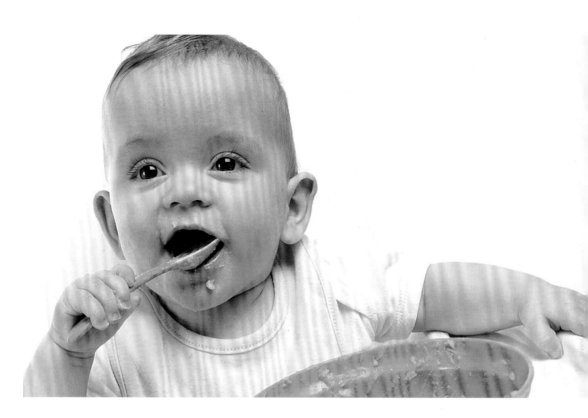

- B$_{12}$: Eggs, cheese, textured vegetable protein, fortified foods, such as breakfast cereals and yeast extract.
- Iron: Beans, lentils, leafy green vegetables, dairy products, fortified breakfast cereals, dried fruit, brown rice, and whole-grain bread.
- Zinc: Nuts, seeds, dairy products, beans, lentils, whole grains, and yeast extract.

SELF-FEEDING

Many babies like to feed themselves from an early age, and you may find that your baby tries to grab her feeding spoon from you. This growing sense of independence is not a bad thing and also encourages good hand/eye coordination, while learning to bite and chew helps with speech development. Let her have her own spoon while you continue feeding with a second one—things may get messy, but that's half the fun.

It may take a few months (or years) for your baby to become proficient at feeding herself with a spoon, and most of the meals may end up on the floor or smeared over the highchair instead of in her mouth. Prepare for the mess by putting a plastic sheet or newspaper on the floor and remaining calm about any mishaps. You can help by supplying foods that are easy to scoop up on a spoon, such as mashed potatoes, thick cottage cheese, cooked rice, and cereal. Finger foods (see page 16) and meals cut into manageable chunks instead of being mashed are easier to pick up and may ease any frustration. The more your baby is allowed to use her hands, the sooner she will probably become more accomplished with a spoon. This also allows her to take an active part in mealtimes and she'll begin to enjoy being involved.

	BREAKFAST	Mid Morning Milk (every day)	LUNCH	Mid Afternoon Milk (every day)
MONDAY	Oatmeal with Apricot Pure 61		Sardines on Toast 72	
TUESDAY	Egg Cups 65		Tomato & Tuna Gnocchi 105	
WEDNESDAY	Date & Vanilla Breakfast Yogurt 57		Baked Potato with Hummus & Roasted Red Pepper filling 80	
THURSDAY	Homemade Baked Beans 78 with toast		Ham & Pea Penne 120	
FRIDAY	Golden Crunch 59		Sweet Potato Casserole 102	
SATURDAY	French Toast 64		Muffin Pizzas 87 and vegetable sticks	
SUNDAY	Banana & Strawberry Smoothie 56 with toast and a well-cooked poached egg		Flounder with Roasted Tomatoes 107	

DINNER

Meaty Paella 118

Macaroni & Cheese Leek with Leeks 94

Vegetable Soup with Chicken Dumplings 111

Salmon Sticks with Sweet Potato Fries 109

Turkey Fricassee 117

Meat Balls with Tomato Sauce 124 and rice

Spaghetti with Roasted Butternut Squash 96

DESSERTS

Apple & Cinnamon Compote 133

Banana & Maple Yogurt Ice 130

Quick Berry Bread Pudding 132

Fruit Yogurt Swirls 128

Mango Whip 129

Peach Crisps 136

Strawberry Sundae 131

Bedtime Milk (every day)

STAGE 4: **Family Meals**

As your baby approaches his first birthday, there are fewer occasions when a specially prepared meal is necessary. He can now enjoy most of the foods as the rest of the family with a few exceptions. Joining in with family meals is one way to learn good eating habits, because these are shaped and honed when young. It is also more convenient because there is no need to prepare separate meals. In the selection of recipes, there are many that both you and your baby will enjoy. When you won't be eating together, consider preparing meals (without seasoning) in bulk and freezing them in baby-size portions for future use, but make sure you defrost and reheat the meals thoroughly before serving. Commercially made baby foods also have their place, but don't let them replace homemade meals altogether.

KEEPING PACE WITH YOUR BABY
Coarsely mash, finely chop, grate, or grind meals, because this will help your baby to practice chewing skills, benefit teeth, and aid speech development. It may take a while for your baby to accept foods with a coarser texture but persist, taking things slowly and being as encouraging and positive as possible.

Babies thrive on routine, and, because their energy requirements are high in relation to the size, they require three small meals a day. If convenient, give the main meal of the day at lunchtime, when your bay is alert and not feeling too grouchy. If your baby has started to crawl or is going through a growth spurt, he also may need a couple of healthy snacks between meals to keep energy levels sufficiently high. Unsurprisingly, sugary, salty, high fat and highly processed snacks are not recommended; they are low in nutrients and high in calories.

Never force your baby to eat, because this will only put him off altogether. If you are worried he is not eating enough, talk to your healthcare provider, who will look at your baby's growth chart and weight and will monitor progress; you may well find that your fears are ungrounded and he is continuing to progress well. If he seems active and lively, then he is probably getting enough energy from

SNACKS TO TRY

- Hard-boiled egg

- Sticks or slices of bread or toast

- Rice cakes with yeast extract

- Pita bread with hummus

- Cheese sticks or grated cheese

- Vegetable sticks, cooked or raw

- Slices or large cubes of fruit

- Pieces of dry, sugar-free cereal

- Yogurt

- Dried fruit

- Toast with nut butter (as long as there is no family history of nut allergy)

- Breadsticks with dip

- Strips of cooked chicken

what he is eating. Milk is also considered a food rather than a drink, so if your baby is drinking 2 to 2½ cups (16 to 20 ounces) a day, then he will be getting a range of important nutrients—but remember it is not a meal replacement.

TROUBLE-FREE MEALTIMES

Your baby is unlikely to love every meal he is given, but don't force him to eat if he turns his nose up. Omit the same food or meal for a few days then try giving it to him again—maybe in a different way this time. Teething and general well-being can undoubtedly influence a baby's eating habits, which many parents will attest can frustratingly change on almost a daily basis.

At this stage, many babies also show an increasing desire for independence and may become choosier about what they eat. The more calm you remain, the less likely your baby will use eating as a time to test your patience and the more harmonious mealtimes will be; sometimes this may be easier said than done, but it's well worth a try.

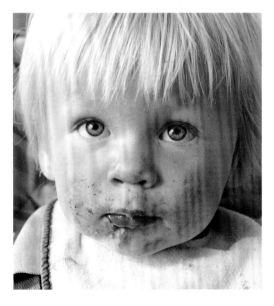

Your baby will probably now be sitting in a high chair or a baby seat attached to the dining table, enabling him to join in with family meals. Self-feeding is an important stage in a baby's development, because it helps hand/eye coordination and encourages independence. Give your baby food with a fairly stiff consistency in a nonslip plastic bowl. Finger foods are also perfect for practicing self-feeding, but you may find that all meals are eaten with his hands at first and this is no bad thing.

MILK

Milk remains an important source of nutrients in your baby's diet for the first year and for many years beyond this; 2 to 2½ cups (16 to 20 ounces) is recommended a day, although some of this amount can be provided by milky puddings and sauces or poured over breakfast cereals. Avoid giving cow, sheep, or goat milk as a drink until your baby is one year old, opting instead for breast, formula, or follow-on milk instead. Continuing to breastfeed ensures that your baby gets milk designed for his needs, so giving other milk may not be needed. If your baby becomes ill and loses his appetite, breastfeeding can keep him well-nourished, giving him important antibodies to tackle bugs, as well as comforting him until he feels better.

OTHER DRINKS

If you haven't done so by now, try weaning your baby off the bottle by introducing a trainer cup with two handles, so he can take sips of water or diluted fresh fruit juice during mealtimes. Drinks from a cup are said to be better for speech development and for his developing teeth. Tea, coffee, soft drinks, sugary fruit drinks, including low-sugar varieties, are not intended for babies and are best avoided.

From one year

Many babies will enjoy family meals by their first birthdays. However, just as you think you have weaning in the bag, it is not uncommon for a child to become more fussy or faddy about food around this age, after having previously wolfed down everything that was offered. This is perfectly normal, and it's good to remember that this is just a stage your toddler is going through; it will not have a long-term detrimental affect on health. Stick to your guns and continue to offer as varied a diet as possible, encompassing a wide range of colors, textures, and flavors. Look at what your toddler eats over a week instead of on a daily basis, and you may find that overall she is eating a good varied diet, despite the occasional meal that remains largely uneaten or the day when she only wants to eat peanut butter sandwiches. Most important, don't panic if your toddler goes through periods of not eating well; you'll no doubt find that she is eating what she needs. Energy requirements increase from years one to three as your toddler continues to grow and becomes more active. Although the need for

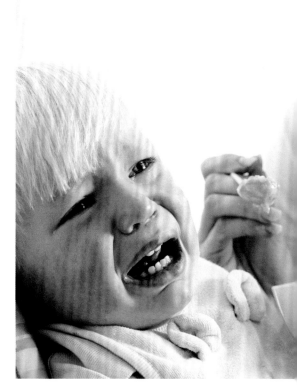

FOCUS ON | sugar and sweets

Most children naturally have a sweet tooth (breast milk and formula milk is sweet, for starters, and babies need this as they feed little and often), but hold off giving your child sugary foods as long as feasible, because sugar cravings are hard to break. Foods made from refined sugar are high in calories, nutritionally poor, will ruin a child's appetite, and lead to tooth decay; what's more, sugary foods often include a fair amount of fat— just think of doughnuts, cookies, and cakes.

Nevertheless, an outright sugar ban can backfire, making sweet treats even more desirable. It may be preferential to avoid overprocessed sugary, artificially colored confections instead of cutting out sugar altogether. Don't resort to foods that replace sugar with artificial sweeteners, because they have been found to cause digestive problems if eaten in large quantities and, in the long-term, they are no better than the refined alternative.

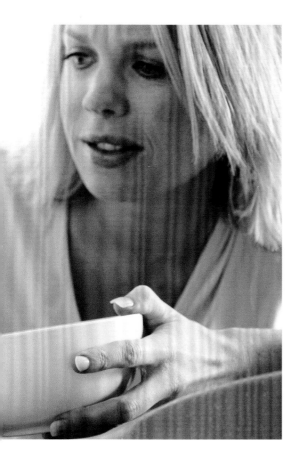

SNACKS TO TRY

- Hard-boiled egg with toast sticks

- Sticks of cheese with apple slices and oat cake

- Toasted cheese muffin

- Chunks of melon with ham

- Tuna mixed with mayonnaise with toasted tortilla triangles

- Hummus and breadsticks

- Rice cake with nut butter

- Mashed banana sandwich

- Pita bread with yeast extract and carrot sticks

- Good-quality meatballs with halved cherry tomatoes

- Dried apple rings

- Fruit muffin

- Plain yogurt with mango

- Slice of fruitcake

- Toasted bagel

- Chunks of fresh fruit

- Raisins or chopped dried fruit

good-quality protein is much the same (two or three servings a day), there is an increased need for all vitamins and minerals, except vitamin D, which is supplied by exposure to sunlight.

KEEP IT HEALTHY

The term "balanced diet" can intimidate even the most nutritionally aware parent, but as long as your child eats a good mixture of foods on a regular basis, then she will get all the nutrients she needs.

A diet high in fiber and low in fat remains unsuitable for children of this age, because this may preclude youngsters being able to obtain all the energy and nutrients they require. Additionally, a diet high in fiber will also reduce

WHAT TODDLERS NEED

The dietary habits of later life are often determined by eating patterns that develop in the early years. If your toddler is picky about her food, as many are, don't be tempted to take the easy option and indulge all her whims. Encourage her to eat as varied a diet as possible.

Carbohydrate/starchy foods
(4–5 servings a day)

Bread, cereals, pasta, rice, and potatoes are excellent sources of energy, fiber, vitamins, and minerals. Carbohydrates should form the main part of every meal, but keep in mind that toddlers find it difficult to digest large amounts of high-fiber foods, such as whole wheat bread and brown rice, so try providing a combination of white and whole-grain carbohydrate foods. If making a fruit crisp, for instance, combine white and whole wheat flour for the topping, and you could also follow this principle if making cookies, cakes, and bread.

Potatoes provide useful amounts of vitamin C, which is found mainly just under the skin, so avoid peeling them if you can. Potatoes with think skins can simply be scrubbed and baked potatoes are also a good source of nutrients. Add sweet potato, rutabaga, or parsnip to mashed potatoes to boost its nutritional value.

Dairy products

Regular milk, cheese, yogurt, and cottage cheese provide protein for growth and development, calcium for teeth, and, together with vitamin D, helps make bones and teeth stronger. Childhood is a crucial time for tooth and bone development and continues to influence bone health in adulthood.

Crème fraîche and Greek plain yogurt make useful alternatives to cream in cooking and are also lower in fat; use them in sauces, soups, pies—both sweet and savory types. (See Milk below.)

Protein foods
(2–3 servings a day)

Meat, poultry, fish, eggs, and beans and other legumes provide rich amounts of vitamins and minerals and are essential for your toddler's growth and development. If she is vegetarian, plan to give her a good mix of protein foods, including beans, lentils, tofu, nuts, and eggs.

Oily fish is the richest source of omega-3 essential fatty acids, which have been found to benefit the brain, eyes, and skin. Research has also shown a correlation between fatty acid levels in children and their intellectual and behavioral performance as youngsters (see page 35). You can give boys up to four servings a week of oily fish, including tuna (canned is not as rich in omega-3 as fresh), salmon, mackerel, herring, sardines, and trout and girls up to two portions. Omega-3 is also found in non-fish sources, such as fortified eggs, drink,s and cereals, walnuts, flaxseed, pumpkin seeds, canola oil, soybeans.

Red meat and liver are rich in iron but cut off any excess fat. Lean, good-quality ground meat can be made into homemade burgers and kofta, or used as a base for pastry or potato-topped pies, pasta sauces, and in stir-fries.

Fruit and vegetables
(5 servings a day)

Whether fresh, frozen, canned, dried, or juiced, fruit and vegetables provide a whole host of vitamins and minerals, especially vitamin C, that are vital for good health. A minimum of five portions a day is recommended and a serving for a toddler is one satsuma, half an apple or banana, five grapes, a floret of broccoli, two teaspoons of peas or carrots, or one tomato. A small glass of fresh fruit juice also counts.

It probably won't come as much of a surprise to find out that most children do not eat enough fresh produce, and the majority of parents will have experienced the struggle to get their children to eat their greens.

Try presenting fruit and vegetables in different ways. For example, many children turn their nose up at cooked vegetables, but will gladly eat them raw, including sticks of cucumber, carrot, and red bell pepper. Vegetables sticks are good for dunking into dips so serve them with nutritious guacamole or hummus (see pages 16 and 70) and you'll double the health benefits. Alternatively, incorporate vegetables into fritters or potato cakes, or if the going gets really tough, disguise pureed vegetables into sauces, stews, soups, and pies. A love of fruit is perhaps easier to encourage, but again maintain the interest with different types and presenting them in various ways.

the amount of minerals absorbed, including valuable iron and calcium. Likewise, children need a certain amount of fat for normal growth and development. Not all fat is bad, and it has an important role to play in transporting vitamins A, D, E, and K through the body. Unsaturated fat is found in vegetables oils, oily fish, and soft margarine and is an important contributor to good health.

Try to provide a good mix of high-energy, nutrient-dense foods based on the food groups on these pages on a daily basis (obviously, the range of foods eaten will vary depending on special diets, eating preferences, and the presence of food intolerances):

SNACKS
Toddlers have high energy requirements for their size; consequently, small, frequent meals plus two to three healthy snacks are necessary for a child of this age, who does not have a large enough stomach to cope with three large meals a day. You'll probably find that your child will need a snack midmorning, midafternoon, and maybe prebedtime. Some children love to graze, take advantage of this by offering healthy snacks, turning them into mini-meals instead of opting for sugary, salty, or fatty processed foods. However, it's also important for children to enjoy main meals and constant snacking can deter them from doing this.

MILK
Regular cow, sheep, or goat milk can be given to children over the age of 12 months as a main drink. Your child still requires 2 to 2½ cups (16 to 20 ounces) milk a day, although some of this can be provided by milky puddings and sauces, or poured over breakfast cereals. Aim for your child to give up a bottle by one year old and to move on to a cup of milk.

While you may still be breastfeeding, it is no longer necessary to offer formula or follow-on milk, although you can continue to do so if you feel your child is not eating well or you are

	BREAKFAST	Breakfast Milk	LUNCH
MONDAY	Golden Crunch 59 with milk and chopped apple		Miso Noodle Soup 85
TUESDAY	French Toast 64 and Homemade Baked Beans 78		Mexican Rice 100
WEDNESDAY	Oatmeal with Apricot Puree 61		Sardines on Toast 72
THURSDAY	Boiled egg and Homemade Baked Beans 78		Halloumi & Pita Salad 77
FRIDAY	Tomato & Egg Scramble 63		Tuna Tortilla Melt 92
SATURDAY	Mini Banana Pancakes 66		Baby Falafel Burgers 89
SUNDAY	Banana & Strawberry Smoothie 56 with Potato Cakes with Beans 67	Milk in smoothie	Mozzarella Tortilla Package 90

DINNER

Roasted Sausages & Potatoes 119

Barbecue Chicken with Coleslaw 112

Creamy Broccoli Pasta Casserole 97

Pork with Fruity Couscous 121

Indian Lentil Soup 104
with rice

Turkey Fricassee 117

Creamy Fish Casserole 108

DESSERTS

Apple, Plum & Oaty Crisp 141

Carrot Cake Square 138

Mixed Fruit Compote 133
with Greek yogurt

Strawberry Yogurt Ice 131

Mango Whip 129

Apple & Cinnamon Compote 133
with ice cream

Lemon Syrup Cakes 139

Bedtime Milk (every day)

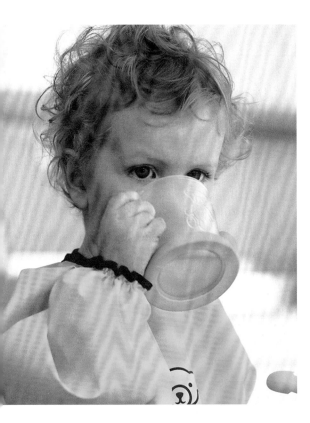

concerned that she is not getting the range of nutrients needed. Low-fat milk can be introduced after your child is two, as long as she is eating well. Skim milk is not recommended for children under five years of age, because it does not provide enough energy and vitamin A for a growing child.

DRINKS

Water is always the best drink option for children, but diluted fresh fruit juice provides vitamin C and if served alongside a meal containing iron, it can help absorption of this mineral. However, even fruit juice contains natural sugars, so avoid giving it to your child other than at mealtimes to prevent damage to her teeth, since the longer a sugary drink is in contact with teeth, the more damage it can do.

Soft drinks and beverages containing caffeine are best avoided, because they are high in sugar, a source of empty calories, and nutritionally poor. They also fill children up, affecting their appetite for meals. Water is the best option between meals.

SUPPLEMENTS

It is recommended that between the ages of one to five years, a liquid supplement of vitamin D should be given unless your infant is eating a good varied diet containing these nutrients and exposure to sunlight is sufficient. These should be continued until your child is five if she is a poor eater or does not have much exposure to sunlight.

FOCUS ON | iron

Iron deficiency is not uncommon in children, so try to give a food or drink rich in vitamin C, such as fruit juice or vegetables, at the same time as an iron-rich food, because it will help the absorption of this mineral.

Don't give tea and coffee to young children, especially at mealtimes; not only do they contain caffeine, but they interfere with the amount of iron absorption. Because iron is more difficult to absorb from nonmeat sources, if your child is vegetarian, opt to give her foods containing iron everyday, such as beans, lentils, green leafy vegetables, dried fruit, particularly apricots and raisins, as well as fortified breakfast cereals.

From Two Years

As your toddler becomes more active, the more calories he will require to give him the energy needed. Encourage your child to eat a variety of foods so he gets a wide range of nutrients (see Keep it Healthy, page 27).

Work on establishing a regular eating pattern based on three meals plus two to three snacks a day. Some children continue to dislike lumps in their food, so chopping or grinding food may make it more acceptable. Alternatively, finger foods are a great way of encouraging your toddler to chew foods and to enjoy those with a coarser texture.

Your toddler may now attend a nursery or other childcare center, and this can come with its own challenges and peer pressure. You may be fortunate to find one that makes its own healthy lunches and snacks, but standards can vary, so talk to other parents and get some feedback about meals. Some childcare centers are open to parents providing their own packed lunches, drinks, and snacks and this may be a welcome option.

GOOD EATING HABITS

Your child is becoming increasingly aware of the world around him, and with this comes a new sense of independence and free will, with both its positive and not so positive side effects, but studies show parents who instill good eating habits from an early age will probably see the benefits in their children long term. Points to consider include:

- Don't get hung up on good eating manners just yet; there's plenty of time for that. Your toddler will continue to make a mess when he eats—crumbs become a way of life. While, ideally, you would like him to eat with a fork or spoon, fingers or hands will continue to be much in use.
- While it's not always feasible for the whole family to eat together, you will reap the benefits when you do, even if you manage

communal mealtimes only at weekends. Eating together encourages talk and discussion between parents and children and gets them away from the TV screen. Children also learn good eating habits from their parents, so make sure you eat up your greens.

- Be patient and persevere. If you manage to persuade your child to try even a mouthful of food, you are making progress, and he may find he likes it after all. Research shows that children acquire a taste for foods over time and it takes an average of ten "tastes" for a child to accept new foods. The theory is that if a parents can persuade their child to eat just one mouthful of carrots on ten occasions, he will learn to like them.
- Attempts to encourage your child to eat healthy foods can be helped if you make food

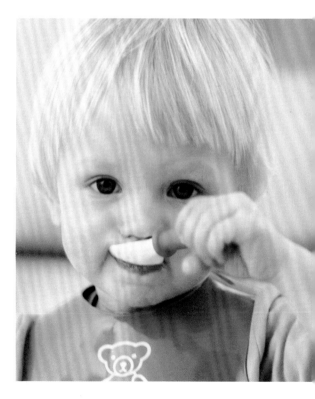

exciting—this doesn't mean that you have to spend hours making faces out of ingredients but keep in mind different colors, textures, and shapes when planning a meal. Interesting or colorful plates, bibs, cutlery, and mats can also make a difference, as can introducing a theme. Steamed vegetables are brighter in color than boiled, while fresh vegetables have an appealing crunchy texture. Imaginative and attractive presentation can usually make the difference between a child eating or refusing a meal.

- Many parents fall into the trap of believing children prefer bland or so-called "children's food." In fact, a study has found that children like stronger flavous than once thought and will happily try chili, stir-fries, and curries, for example, if encouraged.
- Even if you have managed to keep your child away from sugar until now, it will become increasingly more difficult as he becomes older, interacts with other children, and is more aware of children-oriented brands with their brightly colored cartoon

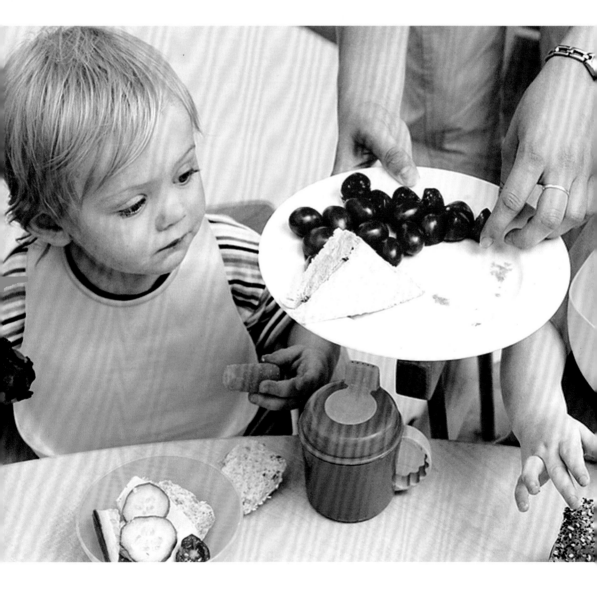

character packaging. Everything in moderation seems to work for most parents, but opt for the ones with the least amount of colors, additives, and preservatives.

- One of the best ways to get your child interested in food is to teach him to cook or at least become involved in the preparation of a meal, even if it's as simple as a quick stir of a sauce or pouring some cereal into a bowl.
- Similarly, get your child involved in food shopping; allow him to choose from healthy options, weigh fresh produce, or unpack.

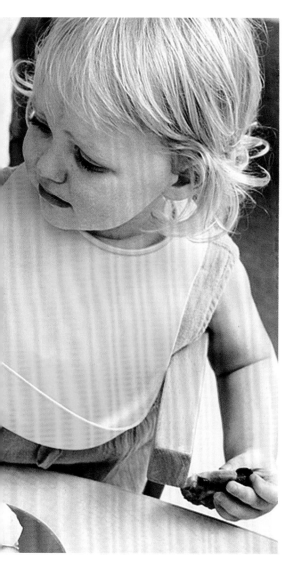

FUSSY EATERS

All children go through stages of picky eating, and appetites can be equally unpredictable—a fact confirmed by the majority of parents. But how do you encourage your child to eat what he is given, and what do you do if he refuses to eat? Perhaps, predictably, there are no easy answers, but the following tips should help you with those more challenging times:

- Forcing your child to eat is a no-win situation for the both of you. Conflict and tension serve only to make the situation more difficult and may lead to your child using mealtimes as a way of seeking attention. It can be incredibly frustrating if your child does not eat a meal that you have lovingly prepared but children are remarkably clever at picking up on the anxieties of their parents and may well tune into your own frustrations about their not eating.
- Gently coax or offer plenty of encouragement to try just a mouthful or a "no thank you bite"; sometimes this is enough for him to be persuaded to eat the rest of the meal.
- Praise your child as much as possible, even if he eats just the one mouthful.
- If encouragement and coaxing don't work, take the food away but don't offer an alternative, however hard this may be. It's important that a child gets used to eating what he is given and does not expect alternatives if he doesn't like the first option.
- Don't make portions too large, because this can be off-putting for a child; you can give him seconds if a meal is eaten up.
- Peer pressure can work both ways. Invite a friend of your child's who you know to be a good eater to lunch. Children often learn by example, and if they see their peers eating up, it may encourage them to do the same.
- Making eating fun. Picnics, even if it is only a cloth arranged on the floor, or a theme based on a favorite game or book can be a real winner.

- Sticker charts can be unbelievably successful and are a simple way of encouraging children to try new foods, especially unfamiliar fruit and vegetables.
- It may be easier said than done, but don't fall into the trap of bribing your child with a dessert or candy.
- Compromise is sometimes the only option. Combine foods you know your child likes with ones previously untried or previously rejected; you may find that new combinations are enough to encourage your child to try new things.

WEIGHT ISSUES

The incidence of obesity in many parts of the world is rising, and unfortunately children are not immune from what is being called an epidemic. The prevalence of obesity has more than doubled among both adults and children living in the United States since the 1970s. Fgures published in 2014 show that almost one of every four children between two and five years old and one of every three school-age children are overweight or obese. The figures were higher among those living in the South. When looking at ethnic groups, the figures tend to be higher among African-American and Hispanic children than in white children. It is also now known that obese mothers tend to have babies who become obese.

Many experts blame the rise in obesity on the growing presence of fast-food outlets, advertising, and the overwhelming choice of cakes, cookies, candy, ice cream, potato chips, snacks, and soft drinks in the stores. While this hasn't helped the situation, lifestyle also has a role to play. With the increasing popularity of computer games and television, children are becoming less and less physically active, so are not burning the calories they have consumed.

However, there could be other reasons for a child being overweight that are not as simple as overeating or inactivity, so it's advisable to consult your doctor before putting your child on any type of diet that could restrict nutritional intake if not handled correctly. Most fat babies will start to thin down when they begin to crawl or walk and become normal-weight toddlers, but a few remain overweight. The best way to prevent a child from becoming fat is to breastfeed exclusively for six months and to teach good eating habits early on; prevention is much easier than cure. Try to stick to a routine of three meals a day plus two to three healthy snacks. Many children are grazers, but constant nibbling makes them

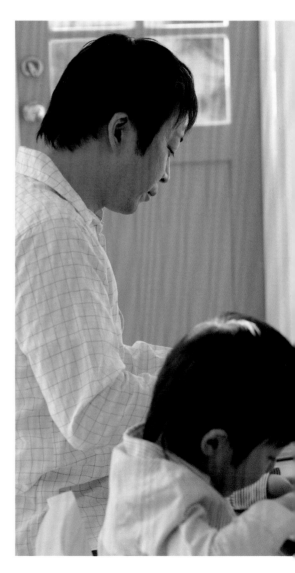

less likely to enjoy a proper meal. Young children should not be put on weight-reduction diets unless advised by a qualified healthcare provider. However, developing a healthy family approach to food and exercise is important in weight management.

MILK

If your child eats well and has a varied, balanced diet, then it is possible, but not necessary, to switch to low-fat milk after two years of age. Skim milk, however, is not recommended before five years, because it does not provide enough energy and nutrients for your growing child.

DRINKS

Many children don't drink enough and will easily go for hours without drinking. Proper hydration helps the brain function at its best, so make sure your child drinks plenty of water, not dehydrating sugary soft drinks. Dehydration can affect concentration as well as the transportation of nutrients around the body.

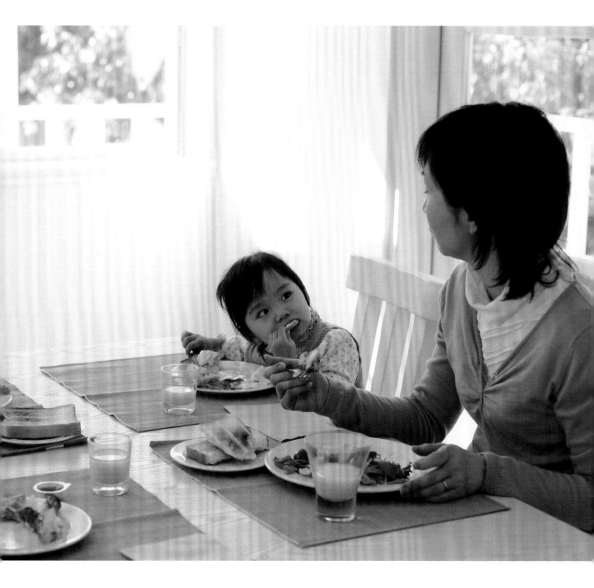

	BREAKFAST	LUNCH
MONDAY	Seedy Banana Breakfast 60	Quick & Easy Sausage Rolls 93 with Vegetable Sticks 101
TUESDAY	Egg Cups 65	Mexican Rice 100
WEDNESDAY	Oatmeal with Apricot Puree 61	Pea Soup 84 with bread
THURSDAY	Ham & Egg Cups 64 with broiled tomatoes	Mini Quiches 88 with Country Garden Salad 76
FRIDAY	Golden Crunch 59 with milk and chopped strawberries	Baby Falafel Burgers 89
SATURDAY	Date & Vanilla Breakfast Yogurt 57 with toast and Three-Nut Butter 58	Vegetable Sticks 101 with steamed vegetables
SUNDAY	Breakfast Omelet 62 and beans	Roasted Red Pesto Chicken 114

DINNER

Pesto & Pea Risotto 99

Ham & Pea Penne 120

Turkey Patties with Pineapple Relish 116

Tomato & Tuna Gnocchi 105

Flounder with Roasted Tomatoes 107

Chinese Beef with Noodles 127

Salmon Frittata 110

DESSERTS

Merry Berry Cobbler 140

Oat Cookie 135
with fruit

Sticky Date Cake 137

Fruit Yogurt Swirls 128

Peach Crisps 136

Quick Berry Bread Pudding 132

Sticky Date Cake 137

Bedtime Milk (every day)

ABOUT THE RECIPES

The recipes have been designed to appeal to children of all ages, and each comes with a recommended age that relates to the suitability of the ingredients used. All First Foods are suitable for babies from six months. Treat these age recommendations as a general guide, because babies progress at different rates. Some may start on purees and then progress to more complex dishes in a few weeks, while others take a little longer. You know your baby best, so please do not feed him something before you think he is ready; however, try to make sure he eats some iron-rich foods (see page 11) from six months, because stores of the mineral deplete from this age.

Use your common sense to serve the dish best suited to your baby's stage of development—pureed, mashed, ground, or chopped.

Many of the main meals have been created for a family of four—two children, two adults—to eat together, but storing suggestions are given if you want to freeze or chill portions for future serving. Some of the recipes contain added sweeteners, but the amount per portion is minimal.

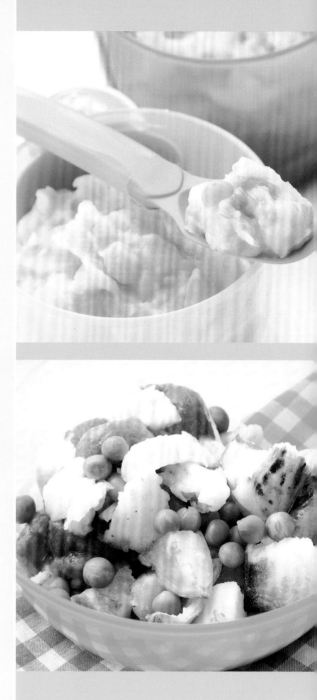

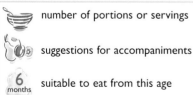

number of portions or servings

suggestions for accompaniments

6 months   suitable to eat from this age

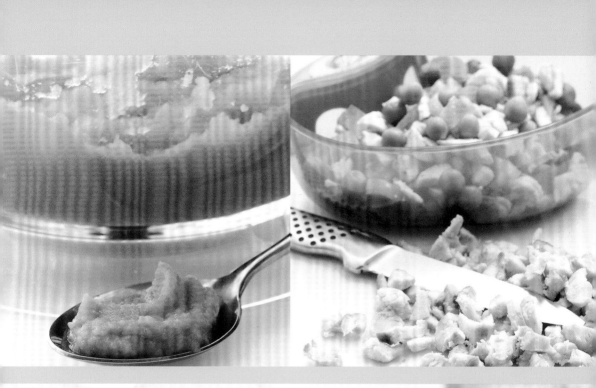

RECIPES

These recipes make excellent starter meals for your baby—all are suitable from the age of six months. They have been intentionally kept simple to enable your baby to try a "taster" of solids and become gradually accustomed to eating.

To begin with, there are a selection of single-ingredient—fruit or vegetable—purees. These are followed by mixed ingredient purees, ranging from simple vegetable and fruit combinations to those incorporating pasta and grains. The single ingredient purees can also be combined to introduce variation. There's also a range of dessert purees.

The portion sizes are a basic guide, and you will probably find that your baby will eat only a few teaspoons (if that) at first. The remainder—not leftovers —can be stored in the refrigerator for a day or you can make double the quantity and freeze in individual portions.

BABY RICE CEREAL

There are many commercial versions of baby rice cereal in the stores, but it's just as easy to make your own. Mix with breast milk or formula milk to make a smooth, thin puree. Baby rice cereal can also be used as a base to mix with fruit and vegetable purees.

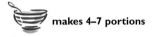 **makes 4–7 portions**

INGREDIENTS

¼ cup white short-grain rice

1 Put the rice into a strainer and rinse under cold running water. Transfer to a saucepan and add enough cold water to cover. Bring to a boil, stir, then reduce the heat.

2 Cover the pan with a lid and simmer for 10–15 minutes, until the water has been absorbed and the grains are tender.

3 Puree the rice in a blender with enough breast or formula milk to make a smooth, runny puree.

STORAGE TIP

Baby rice cereal is suitable for freezing, but make sure it has completely defrosted and is heated through until piping hot to avoid any risk of contamination. Check the temperature before serving.

BANANA PUREE

This makes a perfect first food and is simple to prepare. Make sure you use an especially ripe banana, because it will be much easier on your baby's digestive system.

Remove the skin and put the banana into a bowl. Mash with a fork until as smooth as possible. Add a little boiled water or breast or formula milk to make a thin puree, if necessary.

STORAGE TIP
Unsuitable for freezing

makes 1 portion

INGREDIENTS
½ banana

APPLESAUCE

Apple goes well with baby rice cereal—either homemade or store-bought—and when your baby is ready, it is excellent combined with pureed meat and vegetables.

1 Wash, peel, core, and finely chop the apple. Put the apple into a saucepan with the water and bring to a boil. Reduce the heat and simmer, half-covered, for 5–8 minutes, until tender.

2 Transfer the apple to a blender and puree until smooth, adding a little of the cooking water, if necessary.

VARIATION
Pear can be prepared in the same way as apple. It is an excellent first food, particularly because it is one of the least allergenic of foods. If the pear is nice and ripe, it can simply be peeled, cored, and mashed.

makes 2–3 portions

INGREDIENTS
1 sweet, crisp apple
2 tablespoons water

MELON PUREE

Any variety of melon can be given uncooked to your baby, but make sure it is ripe and juicy.
Wash the skin of the melon before cutting into it. It may be necessary to steam the melon
if it's not entirely ripe.

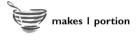 **makes 1 portion**

INGREDIENTS

1 small wedge melon

Scoop out the seeds from the melon, then cut away the flesh from
the skin. Puree to a smooth consistency; it's unlikely you will need
to add any water, because melon has a high water content.

VARIATION
Mango and papaya also make great first foods, simply prepare them
as above.

PREPARATION TIP
If the melon is ripe enough, you will probably be able to mash it
with a fork or pass through a strainer until smooth.

PEACH PUREE

There is nothing nicer than a ripe, juicy peach, and it makes a delicious puree. Nectarines,
plums, and apricots are suitable alternatives. It's wise to make a larger quantity, especially if the
fruit is in season, and freeze in portions for later use.

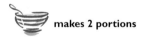 **makes 2 portions**

INGREDIENTS

1 ripe peach
2 tablespoons water

1 Quarter the peach, removing the pit in the center, then put it
into a saucepan with the water. Bring to a boil, then simmer
the fruit for 8–10 minutes.

2 Remove the peach from the cooking water and when cool
enough to handle, peel off the skin.

3 Transfer the peach to a blender and puree until smooth,
adding a little boiled water, if necessary.

STORAGE TIP
Suitable for freezing

CARROT PUREE

The wonderful color and natural sweetness of carrot makes it a popular first food.

1 Scrape or peel the carrot, then cut into bite-size pieces. Put the carrot into a saucepan with the water. Bring to a boil and cook for 10 minutes, until tender.

2 Put the carrot into a blender with a little of the cooking water and blend until a smooth puree.

VARIATION
When your baby is familiar with carrot, try pureeing it with cooked potato or butternut squash.

STORAGE TIP
Suitable for freezing

makes 2–3 portions

INGREDIENTS
1 carrot
2 tablespoons water

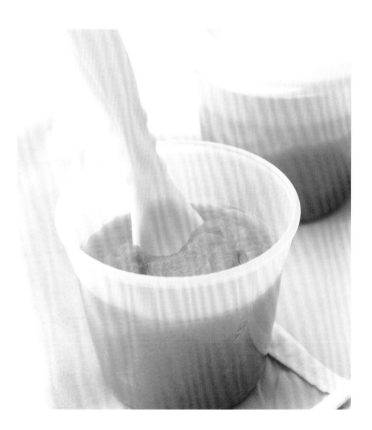

AVOCADO PUREE

Avocadoes are rich in nutrients and beneficial oils; they also make a perfect quick meal, because they do not require cooking. Make sure you use a ripe avocado and prepare it just before serving, because it discolors soon after cutting. You could omit the yogurt, if preferred.

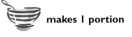 **makes I portion**

INGREDIENTS

½ small avocado
2 teaspoons plain yogurt
(optional)

1 Cut the avocado in half lengthwise and remove the pit. Scoop out the flesh into a bowl, using a teaspoon.

2 Mash the avocado with a fork until smooth and creamy. Mix in the yogurt and stir thoroughly until combined. Serve immediately.

STORAGE TIP

Not suitable for freezing. Squeeze fresh lemon juice over the remaining half of avocado to prevent it from discoloring. Keep the avocado in the refrigerator for use the following day.

SWEET POTATO PUREE

Sweet potato makes a nutritious puree and a useful base for other mixed purees. The orange-fleshed ones are richer in vitamin C and beta-carotene than those with a white flesh. Blend with breast or formula milk for a creamy textured puree.

 makes 4–6 portions

INGREDIENTS

I small, orange-fleshed
sweet potato

1 Peel the sweet potato and cut into bite-size chunks. Cover with water, bring to a boil, and cook for 10–15 minutes, until tender.

2 Drain the potatoes and transfer to a blender with a little breast or formula milk to make a smooth, creamy puree.

VARIATION

Yams and potatoes can also be prepared in the same way. When your baby is familiar with single-ingredient purees, you could combine these with a little grated cheese, cooked poultry, meat, fish, beans or other legumes, or other vegetables.

MIXED PUREES

Once your baby is familiar with a selection of single-ingredient purees, increase the range of flavors by combining different foods together. You could also increase the texture from thin, runny ones to more coarsely textured purees or even mashed or ground foods.

PEA & ZUCCHINI PUREE

Zucchini have a light, slightly watery texture and combine well with more fiber-rich peas. This can be mixed with potato, too.

1 Trim and slice the zucchini; there is no need to peel it. Steam or boil the zucchini and peas for 3 minutes, until tender.

2 Mash until a coarse puree or transfer to a blender and puree until smooth, adding a little of the cooking water, if necessary.

VARIATION
Instead of the zucchini, use 3 small florets of broccoli. Steam for 5 minutes before adding the peas, and cook for another 3 minutes, until tender. Mash until a coarse puree or transfer to a blender and puree until smooth, adding a little of the cooking water, if necessary.

makes 2–4 portions

INGREDIENTS

1 zucchini
Small handful of
  frozen peas

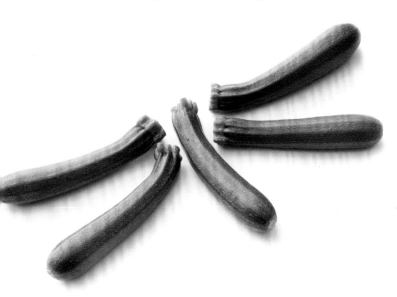

LEEK, POTATO & CORN PUREE

This baby-friendly version of the classic corn chowder makes an excellent flavorsome puree. Blend with breast or formula milk for a creamy texture.

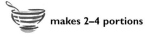

makes 2–4 portions

INGREDIENTS

1 Yukon gold or
  russet potato
½ small leek
3 tablespoons canned
  no-sugar and no-
  sodium corn kernels

1 Peel the potato and cut into bite-size chunks. Wash the leek, remove the tough outer layer, then slice thinly.

2 Steam or boil the potatoes and leek for 12–15 minutes, adding the corn 3 minutes before the end of the cooking time. Cook until the vegetables are tender.

3 Transfer the vegetables to a blender and blend with a little breast or formula milk until pureed.

VARIATION

To increase the nutritional value or this mixed vegetable puree, you could add a protein food, such as grated cheese, cooked skinless chicken, white fish, or a hard-boiled egg.

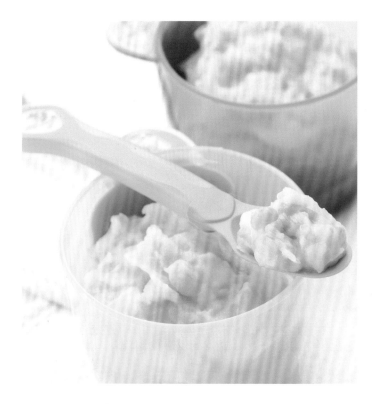

SQUASH, PARSNIP & APPLE PUREE

Rich in vitamin C, this nourishing puree would also taste delicious as an accompaniment to roasted pork. Puree or mash, depending on desired consistency.

1 Put the squash and parsnip into a saucepan and cover with water. Bring to a boil, then reduce the heat and simmer for 10 minutes.

2 While the vegetables are cooking, wash, peel, core, and dice the apple and then add to the pan. Cook for another 5 minutes, until everything is tender.

STORAGE TIP
Suitable for freezing

makes 4–6 portions

INGREDIENTS

½ cup washed, peeled, seeded, and diced butternut squash
1 small parsnip
1 sweet, crisp apple

OAT & VEGETABLE PUREE

Oats give extra substance to this vegetable puree.

1 Put the oats into a small saucepan, cover with water, and bring to a boil. Reduce the heat and simmer, covered, for 4–5 minutes, until soft and creamy. Stir the oats occasionally to prevent them from sticking to the bottom of the pan.

2 While the oats are cooking, steam the leeks for 10 minutes, until tender. Drain any excess water from the oats, if necessary, and add the leeks, tomato, and corn kernels to the pan with 2 tablespoons milk (breast, formula, or cow).

3 Add the butter to the pan and stir until heated through. Puree or mash, depending on the desired consistency.

VARIATION
Try adding two tablespoons cooked and ground chicken or beef.

makes 4–6 portions

INGREDIENTS

2 tablespoons rolled oats
1 small leek, finely chopped
2 tablespoons canned no-sugar and no-sodium corn kernels
1 tomato, skinned, seeded, and chopped
small pat of unsalted butter or margarine

VEGETABLE & PASTA STEW

This is a nutritious combination of vegetables, pasta, and beans, which provides a good range of vitamins and minerals.

makes 4–6 portions

INGREDIENTS

1 tablespoon olive oil

1 small onion

1 small carrot, scrubbed and finely diced

½ teaspoon dried oregano

1¼ cups water

⅓ cup tomato puree

2 oz small soup pasta

¼ cup canned no-sodium, no-sugar cranberry or pinto beans, drained and rinsed

½ cup finely chopped baby spinach

2 tablespoons freshly grated Parmesan cheese

1 Heat the olive oil in a medium saucepan. Add the onion and carrot and sauté, stirring, for 10 minutes, until softened.

2 Add the oregano, water, and tomato puree. Bring to a boil, then reduce the heat and simmer, covered, for 10 minutes.

3 Next, stir in the pasta and beans, return the soup to a boil, and simmer until the pasta is tender, stirring occasionally. Add the spinach and cook for another 2 minutes.

4 Stir in the Parmesan and puree, mash, or chop, depending on the desired consistency; you may need to add a little more boiled water, if pureeing.

VARIATION

Instead of the pasta and beans, add 2 tablespoons red split lentils in step 2 and cook for 20 minutes, adding more water, if necessary. When the lentils are tender, stir in the spinach and cook according to the recipe.

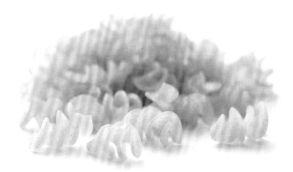

CHICKEN WITH TOMATO RICE

This makes a satisfying and tasty addition to your baby's diet. You could try a combination of white and brown rice to increase nutrient levels.

1 Preheat the broiler to medium-high and line the broiler pan with aluminum foil. Put the chicken into the broiler pan and brush with oil. Broil for 6–8 minutes each side, until cooked through and there is no trace of pink.

2 While the chicken is cooking, put the rice and diced tomatoes into a saucepan with the water. Bring to a boil and add the oregano, carrot, and beans.

3 Reduce the heat, cover, and simmer for 15–20 minutes, or until the water has been absorbed and the vegetables are tender.

4 Finely chop the chicken and mix into the rice, then puree or grind until the desired consistency; you may need to add a little extra boiled water.

VARIATION
In place of the chicken, broil a fillet of white fish for 10–15 minutes, depending on the thickness. Remove the skin and any bones, then flake the fish and stir into the rice.

STORAGE TIP
Suitable for freezing. If freezing the rice, make sure it is completely defrosted before reheating. Heat through completely to avoid any risk of food contamination.

makes 6–8 portions

INGREDIENTS

4 oz skinless, boneless chicken breast, cut into strips
olive oil, for brushing
⅓ cup white rice
⅓ cup canned diced tomatoes
¾ cup water
½ teaspoon dried oregano
1 small carrot, scrubbed and finely diced
3 fine green beans, thinly sliced

MASHED BEANS & VEGETABLES

This is a nutritious combination of vegetables, pasta, and beans, which provides a good range of vitamins and minerals.

makes 4 portions

INGREDIENTS

- 1 Yukon gold or russet potato, peeled
- 1 beet or parsnip, peeled
- 1 teaspoon olive oil
- 1½ tablespoons unsalted butter
- ¼ cup no-sodium, no-sugar baked beans
- 2 tablespoons shredded cheddar cheese

1 Cut the potato and beet or parsnip, into bite-size pieces and put into a saucepan. Cover with water and bring to a boil.

2 Reduce the heat and simmer for 15–20 minutes, until tender. Drain and puree or mash the vegetables with the olive oil and butter.

3 Heat the beans gently, then mash. Stir the beans into the mashed vegetables with the cheese.

VARIATION
Replace the cheese with the yolk of one hard-boiled egg. Peel the egg, discard the white, then mash the yolk into the beans and vegetables.

STORAGE TIP
Suitable for freezing.

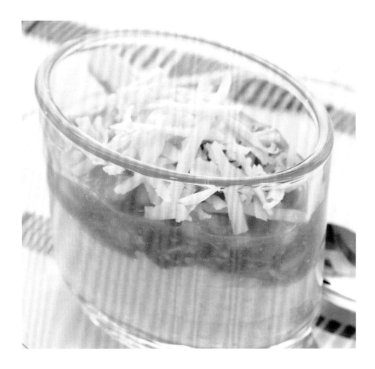

DESSERTS

Even small babies have a natural "sweet tooth," which can be satisfied with a fruit-base dessert. Because the fruit is mixed with yogurt or served iced, the cool temperature and smooth texture can be soothing for babies cutting their first teeth.

DRIED APRICOT PUREE

Dried apricots are a good source of iron, a mineral that is vital especially because a baby's stores begin to diminish from around six months of age. Like other dried fruit, apricots are high in fiber, so it's important that they are given in small amounts. Here, the apricots are mixed with plain yogurt to produce a creamy puree.

1 Wash the apricots and cut them into small pieces. Put the apricots into a saucepan, cover with water, and bring to a boil, then reduce the heat and simmer for 20 minutes until soft.

2 Transfer to a blender and blend until pureed, adding a little of the cooking water, if necessary. Let cool slightly, then mix with the yogurt.

INGREDIENT TIP
Sulfur is commonly used to preserve dried fruit, but is best avoided by those susceptible to asthma, because it is known to exacerbate symptoms. Unsulfured apricots are dark brown in color and have a rich, almost caramel-like flavor.

makes 5–8 portions

INGREDIENTS

10 unsulfured
    dried apricots
3 tablespoons
    plain yogurt

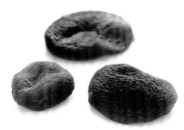

ORCHARD FRUIT YOGURT

It is worth making a larger portion of this stewed fruit for later use. Freeze the fruit mixture, then defrost before mixing with the yogurt.

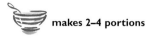 **makes 2–4 portions**

INGREDIENTS

2 plums
1 sweet, crisp apple
2 tablespoons water
¼–⅓ cup yogurt
1 plain cookie (optional)

1 Halve the plums and remove the pit. Peel, core, and chop the apple into bite-size pieces. Put the fruit into a saucepan and add the water.

2 Bring to a boil, then reduce the heat and simmer for 5–8 minutes, until tender. Remove the plum skins, then puree the fruit in a blender or pass through a strainer.

3 Crush the cookie, if using. Mix together the fruit and yogurt and sprinkle with the crushed cookie, if using, before serving.

STORAGE TIP
Cooked fruit is suitable for freezing

BANANA YOGURT CUSTARD

This is the simplest of desserts and would also make a quick breakfast or snack. Make sure the banana is ripe, becuase it will be easier for your baby to digest.

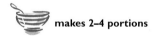 **makes 2–4 portions**

INGREDIENTS

1 small banana, peeled
2 tablespoons plain
  Greek yogurt
3 tablespoons prepared
  custard or vanilla
  pudding

Mash the banana until fairly smooth. Combine the banana, yogurt, and custard, then serve.

VARIATION
Replace the banana with 1 cup hulled strawberries.

STORAGE TIP
Suitable for freezing

FRUIT WHIP

Not only is fresh mango packed with vitamin C, it is delicious pureed. Combine with fromage blanc or yogurt and you have a quick whip that can be served as a breakfast, dessert, or snack.

1 Peel the mango and cut away the flesh from the pit. Puree the fruit or pass through a strainer.

2 Mix together the mango puree and fromage blanc or plain Greek yogurt before serving.

STORAGE TIP
Suitable for freezing

makes 2–4 portions

INGREDIENTS

½ ripe mango
⅓ cup fromage blanc
or plain Greek yogurt

QUICK BANANA ICE CREAM

This speedy ice cream is perfect for soothing sore gums, if your baby is teething.

1 Peel the banana and wrap in plastic wrap. Freeze for about 3 hours, until solid.

2 Remove the banana from the freezer and take off the plastic wrap. Let soften slightly, then mash with a fork.

STORAGE TIP
Suitable for freezing

makes 2 portions

INGREDIENTS

1 banana

BANANA & STRAWBERRY SMOOTHIE

It can sometimes be difficult to get children to eat breakfast, yet a smoothie served in a brightly colored cup may be just the thing to renew interest. It is full of vital nutrients and provides much needed energy for the morning ahead. The fruit provide vitamin C and magnesium, while the milk and yogurt contain calcium, all essential for healthy skin, bones, and teeth.

1–2 child-size servings

toast and a boiled egg for a nutritionally complete breakfast

INGREDIENTS

1 small banana, sliced

3 strawberries, hulled and halved, if large

2 tablespoons plain Greek yogurt

¼ cup milk (breast, formula, cow, or alternative)

Put all the ingredients into a blender and blend until thick, smooth, and creamy, then pour the smoothie into cups or glasses, adding more milk, if necessary. (Straw optional.)

SERVING TIP

You could freeze the smoothie in a lidded container to make a simple yogurt ice, or alternatively, omit the milk and serve as a natural fruit yogurt.

STORAGE TIP

Smoothies don't generally keep longer than a day. Store any surplus smoothie in an airtight container in the refrigerator. Add a squeeze of lemon juice to help prevent the banana from discoloring.

6 months

DATE & VANILLA BREAKFAST YOGURT

This thick and creamy fruit yogurt is a nourishing and energy-boosting blend of protein and slow-release carbohydrates, making it an excellent start to the day.

1 Put the dates and ⅔ cup of water into a medium saucepan. Bring to a boil, then reduce the heat. Put a lid on and simmer for 10 minutes, until the dates are soft. Let cool.

2 Put the dates and any remaining water, yogurt, vanilla extract, and milk into a blender. Blend until smooth and creamy. Spoon into a bowl.

SERVING TIP

You could freeze the yogurt in a lidded container to make a simple yogurt ice, or alternatively add extra milk (breast, formula, cow, or alternative) to make a nutritious smoothie.

STORAGE TIP

Store any surplus in an airtight container in the refrigerator for up to three days.

2 child-size servings

sticks of toasted fruit bread for dipping in

INGREDIENTS

⅓ cup coarsely chopped, pitted dried dates

¼ cup plain Greek yogurt

½ teaspoon vanilla extract

¼ cup milk (breast, formula, cow, or alternative)

6 months

APRICOT & PRUNE FRUIT SPREAD

A healthier alternative to commercial preserves and jellies, this contains considerably more fruit and less sugar, and is an excellent source of vitamins and minerals, especially iron.

 makes about 1 cup

spread thinly on plain or toasted bread, muffins, or bagels

INGREDIENTS

1 cup coarsely chopped unsulfured dried apricots
1 cup coarsely chopped dried prunes
2 cups water

1   Put the apricots and prunes into a nonmetallic saucepan. Cover with 1¾ cups water and bring to a boil. Reduce the heat, cover, and simmer for 45 minutes, until the fruit is soft, swollen, and almost caramelized.

2   Transfer the cooked fruit to a blender or food processor and blend with the remaining water to make a thick puree. Spoon the fruit spread into an airtight jar or container and store in the refrigerator for up to a week.

6+ months

THREE-NUT BUTTER

This homemade butter contains no additives or sugar—unlike many commercial varieties.

8 child-size servings

spread thinly on toast, sticks of pita bread, or bagels

INGREDIENTS

¼ cup shelled almonds
¼ cup cashew nuts
2 tablespoons shelled peanuts
3–4 tablespoons sunflower oil

1   Toast the nuts in a dry skillet for 2–5 minutes. Rub the nuts in a clean dish towel to remove the papery brown covering, if necessary.

2   Transfer the nuts to a food processor or blender and process until finely ground.

3   Pour the oil into the blender or food processor and blend to a coarse paste. Store in an airtight jar or container in the refrigerator for up to a week.

6 months

Note Contains nuts: Avoid serving to babies if there is a history of nut allergy, asthma, hay fever, or eczema within the immediate family. Please consult your pediatrician or healthcare professional.

GOLDEN CRUNCH

It is important to include a good range of essential fatty acids in a child's diet, and the nuts and seeds in this granola provide a nourishing mix of both omega-3 and omega-6 fatty acids. If serving to babies under a year, finely grind the cereal and cook and puree the apricots.

1 Preheat the oven to 275°F. Put the oats, almonds, pecans, and seeds into a large bowl.

2 Heat the oil and maple syrup in a saucepan over medium heat, stirring until melted and mixed together. Stir in the oats, nuts, and seeds, then mix well until they are thoroughly coated.

3 Spoon onto two baking sheets in an even layer and bake in the preheated oven for 25 minutes, turning halfway, until golden and slightly crisp. (The mixture will become crisper as it cools.)

4 Return the cereal to a bowl and mix in the chopped apricots. Let cool, then transfer to an airtight container.

VARIATION

For a special breakfast treat, place two to three slices of banana in the bottom of a tall glass. Top with 1 tablespoon of plain yogurt, followed by 1 teaspoon Golden Crunch (without the dried apricots). Top with another tablespoons of the yogurt and decorate with two to three more slices of banana. Makes 1 child-size serving.

STORAGE TIP

Store Golden Crunch in an airtight jar or container for up to three weeks.

12 child-size servings

pour on milk (breast, formula, cow, or alternative); top with fresh fruit, such as chopped or pureed strawberries, mashed banana, or stewed pear or apple

INGREDIENTS

1 cup rolled oats
⅓ cup slivered almonds
¼ cup coarsely pecans
3 tablespoons sesame seeds
3 tablespoons sunflower seeds
1½ tablespoons sunflower oil
3 tablespoons maple syrup
⅓ cup finely chopped unsulfured dried apricots

8 months

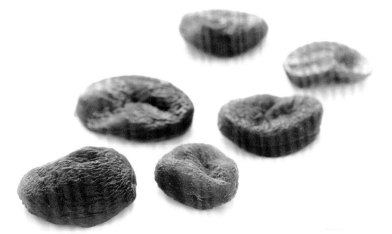

Note Contains nuts (and seeds); avoid serving to babies if there is a history of nut allergy, asthma, hay fever, or eczema within the immediate family. Please consult your pediatrician or healthcare professional.

SEEDY BANANA BREAKFAST

This simple breakfast provides plenty of essential vitamins and minerals. Plain yogurt live has a thick, smooth consistency; bio yogurt with live cultures contains beneficial bacteria that restores equilibrium in the digestive tract.

1–2 child-size servings

with toast

INGREDIENTS

1 tablespoon mixed seeds, such as sunflower, pumpkin, and sesame
1 small banana, mashed
⅓ cup plain yogurt
2 teaspoon maple syrup (optional)

1 Lightly toast the seeds in a dry skillet until just golden, tossing frequently. Transfer them to a grinder and process until finely ground.

2 Mix together the banana and yogurt, then stir in the seeds. Drizzle each serving with the maple syrup, if using.

SERVING TIP
You could make a larger quantity of the ground seed mixture, then stir a spoonful into sauces, soups, burgers, and vegetarian casseroles to enhance their nutritional value.

Note *This breakfast contains seeds; avoid serving to babies if there is a history of nut allergy, asthma, hay fever, or eczema within the immediate family. Please consult your pediatrician.*

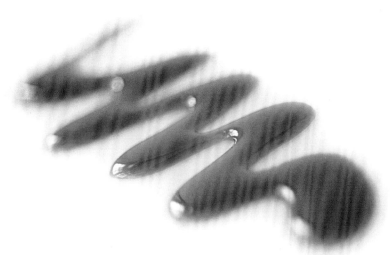

8+ months

OATMEAL WITH APRICOT PUREE

Oatmeal is an excellent breakfast for young children—not only does it taste good, but research has shown that children who eat a carbohydrate-base breakfast, such as oatmeal, have improved concentration and so perform better at school.

1 To make the apricot puree, put the apricots into a saucepan and cover with the water. Bring to a boil, cover the pan, then reduce the heat and simmer for 30 minutes, until the apricots are tender. Put the apricots, along with any water left in the pan, into a blender or food processor and puree until smooth, adding more water, if necessary.

2 To make the oatmeal, put the oats into a saucepan. Add the milk and bring to a boil, stirring occasionally. Reduce the heat and simmer, stirring frequently, for 6 minutes, until smooth and creamy.

3 Pour the oatmeal into a bowl and stir in a large spoonful of the apricot puree.

VARIATION

Dried dates, prunes, and figs make delicious fruit purees and are an excellent source of iron. Use the same method as for the apricot puree and top with a sprinkling of lightly roasted chopped slivered almonds for a delicious, nutritious breakfast, if there is no history of nut allergy within the family.

You could use half milk, half water to make the oatmeal. Instead of the apricot puree, try mashed banana or stewed pear or apple.

1–4 child-size servings (puree serves 4–6)

1 teaspoon honey, if your child is 12 months or older

INGREDIENTS

Apricot puree
1 cup dried apricots
1¼ cups water

Oatmeal
⅔ cup rolled oats
½ cup milk (breast, formula, cow, or alternative) or half milk, half water

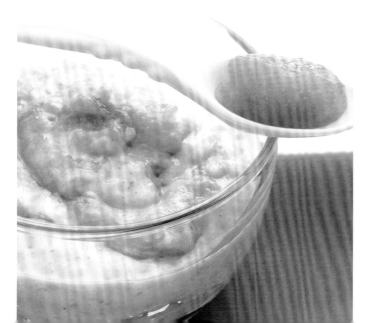

6 months

BREAKFAST OMELET

Children love this complete breakfast in a skillet, which is somewhat similar to an Spanish omelet. It makes a substantial weekend breakfast-cum-brunch, or also a perfect supper dish. If serving to young infants, make sure they are ready to eat finger foods, or you could try mashing the omelet with baked beans.

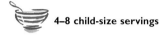 **4–8 child-size servings**

baked beans and toast

INGREDIENTS

3 good-quality link sausages
   (or vegetarian alternative)
4 cooked white round or
   red-skinned potatoes,
   cooled and cut into
   bite-size chunks
6 cherry tomatoes, halved
4 eggs, beaten
sunflower oil, for frying

1 Preheat the broiler to medium-high. Arrange the sausages on an aluminum foil-lined broiler pan, then broil until cooked through and golden. Let cool slightly, then slice into small chunks.

2 Meanwhile, heat a little oil in a medium, heavy skillet with an ovenproof handle. Cook the potatoes until lightly browned all over, then add the tomatoes and cook for another 2 minutes.

3 Arrange the sausages in the skillet so there is an even distribution of potatoes, tomatoes, and sausages.

4 Add a little more oil to the pan if it seems dry. Pour the beaten eggs over the ingredients in the skillet. Cook for 3 minutes without stirring or disturbing the omelet.

5 Place under the preheated broiler for an additional 3 minutes, until the top is just cooked. Serve mashed with beans or cut into wedges and serve with toast.

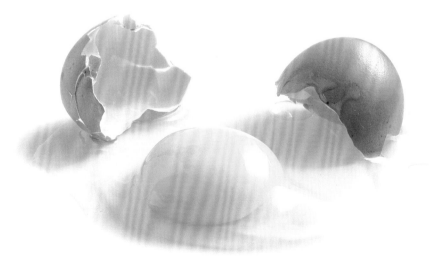

8 months

TOMATO & EGG SCRAMBLE

This simple breakfast or light lunch is a good source of iron and the B vitamins. Make sure the eggs are well-cooked and there is no sign of runniness before serving. If you haven't progressed to finger foods with your baby, omit the bagel until you feel he or she is at the right stage.

1 | Heat the butter in a medium, heavy saucepan. Add the tomatoes and cook for 2 minutes, until softened, stirring occasionally.

2 | Lightly beat the egg with the milk. Pour the mixture into the skillet and, using a wooden spoon, stir constantly to make sure the egg doesn't stick to the bottom of the pan. Continue to cook the egg, stirring, until it is cooked and not runny; this should take about 4 minutes.

3 | Meanwhile, toast and butter the bagel and cut into wedges. Serve with the scrambled egg.

PREPARATION TIP

For babies, you may prefer to peel the tomato beforehand. Make a cross-shape slit in the top of the tomato and put it into boiled water for 1 minute to loosen the skin. Scoop out the tomato with a slotted spoon and peel off the skin; if it refuses to peel, put the tomato back in the water. When skinned, cut the tomato into quarters, scoop out the seeds, and finely chop.

1 child-size serving

toasted bagel along with a glass of orange juice to encourage the absorption of iron from the eggs

INGREDIENTS

1½ tablespoons unsalted butter, plus extra to serve
1 medium tomato, seeded and diced
2 medium eggs
1 tablespoon milk (breast, formula, cow, or alternative)
½ bagel

6 months

FRENCH TOAST

Bread dipped into an egg-and-milk mixture makes great finger food and, for added appeal, cut the bread into fun shapes—diamonds, hearts, or flowers—before dipping into the egg.

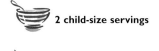 **2 child-size servings**

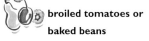 broiled tomatoes or baked beans

INGREDIENTS

1–2 slices of whole-wheat
  or white bread
1 egg, beaten
1 tablespoon milk (breast,
  formula, cow, or alternative)
Butter, for frying

1 | Cut the bread into the desired shapes with pastry cutters or leave as a slice, if preferred. Whisk together the egg and milk in a wide, shallow bowl and dip the bread shapes into the mixture.

2 | Heat some butter in a heavy skillet, place the bread in the pan, and cook, turning once, until the egg has set and is well cooked and golden. Serve immediately.

VARIATION
For a sweet version, prepare and cook as above, but sprinkle with a little sugar and ground cinnamon before serving.

7 months

HAM & EGG CUPS

Eggs make a nutritious start to the day, providing much needed protein, vitamins D and B, and zinc, but for young children, it must be thoroughly cooked; these cups make great finger food.

 4 child-size servings

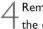 toast and broiled, skinned tomatoes

INGREDIENTS

olive oil, for greasing
4 slices lean ham
4 eggs

1 | Preheat the oven to 400°F. Lightly grease four cups of a deep muffin pan and arrange a slice of ham in each one, overlapping the sides to make it fit and form a "cup" shape.

2 | Trim the top of the ham to make it even, but make sure it is still slightly above the top of the pan.

3 | Crack an egg into each ham-lined muffin cup, then bake for 10 minutes, or until the whites and yolks are firm and set.

4 | Remove from the oven and let cool slightly before removing the cups from the pan.

STORAGE TIP
The cups will keep in the refrigerator for up to two days.

8 months

EGG CUPS

Baby brioche are great for filling with all kinfd of sweet and savory goodies. Scrambled egg makes a great filling and is also a good source of iron and protein. If your baby hasn't progressed to finger foods, omit the brioche until you feel he or she is ready.

1 Preheat the oven to 275°F. Wrap the brioche in aluminum foil and warm in the oven.

2 Meanwhile, heat the butter in a heavy saucepan. When it has melted, add the eggs. Using a wooden spoon, stir constantly to to make sure the egg doesn't stick to the bottom of the pan. Continue to cook the egg, stirring, until the eggs are scrambled thoroughly and not runny; this should take about 4 minutes.

3 Slice off the top of each brioche and scoop out the center. Spoon the scrambled egg into the brioche cups and sprinkle with the chives, if using. Replace the lids of the brioches before serving or, alternatively, cut into strips.

1–2 child-size servings

to serve as finger food, cut the brioche into strips and omit chives

INGREDIENTS

1-2 small brioche rolls
2 eggs, beaten
1 tablespoon unsalted butter
Few snipped chives, to garnish
  (optional)

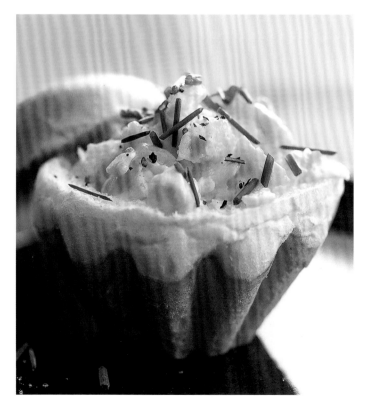

7 months

MINI BANANA PANCAKES

These pancakes make an energizing breakfast and would also make a suitable snack or dessert. Bananas are a good source of potassium, which plays a key role in nerve cell function.

about 10 pancakes
1 pancake will serve an eight month old

fresh fruit and a drizzle of maple syrup

INGREDIENTS

¾ cup all-purpose flour
1 tablespoon sugar
1 teaspoon baking soda
1 egg, lightly beaten
½ cup milk
2 tablespoons plain
   Greek yogurt
1 banana, mashed
Sunflower oil, for frying

1 Sift the flour, sugar, and baking soda into a mixing bowl. Make a well in the center of the flour mixture.

2 Beat the eggs with the milk in a small bowl and gradually pour into the bowl, whisking continuously to avoid any lumps. Add the yogurt and stir to make a smooth and creamy batter. Set the batter aside for 20 minutes, then stir in the banana.

3 Lightly oil a large, heavy skillet and wipe with a folded sheet of paper towel to remove any excess. Heat the pan until hot, then place 2 tablespoons of batter per pancake—you will probably be able to cook three pancakes at a time—in the pan.

4 Cook each pancake for 2–3 minutes, or until the bottom is lightly golden, then turn over and cook for another minute. Place the pancakes on a plate and cover with aluminum foil to keep them warm while you make the remaining pancakes.

5 To serve as finger food, cut into strips. Alternatively, top with banana slices or fruit of choice and maple syrup.

STORAGE TIP
Pancakes freeze well, so you could make larger quantities and keep some for future use; defrost, then wrap in aluminum foil and warm in the oven.

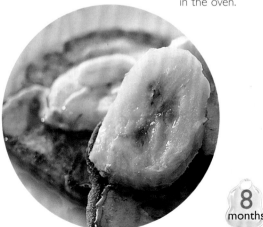

8 months

POTATO CAKES WITH BEANS

A great way of using up leftover mashed potatoes, these mini pancakes can be served on their own or alongside broiled tomatoes, or good-quality sausages or bacon. They also make ideal finger food.

1 Beat together the mashed potatoes and milk in a bowl to make a coarse potato puree.

2 Put the flour and baking powder into a separate bowl, make a well in the center, and add the beaten egg, then gradually add the potato puree. Whisk to make a smooth, creamy, fairly thick batter.

3 Heat a little oil in a large nonstick skillet. Ladle one-quarter of the batter into the pan for each pancake and cook for 2 minutes on each side, until golden. You may have to make the pancakes in batches; if so, keep the finished ones warm while you cook the remaining potato cakes.

4 Warm the baked beans in a saucepan and serve with the potato cakes, which can be cut into sticks, if preferred.

STORAGE TIP
The potato cakes freeze well and will keep for up to three months in a freezer. Make up to step 3, let cool, then freeze in between sheets of wax paper to prevent them from sticking together. Defrost and warm in the oven before serving.

4 cakes
I cake will serve an eight month old
broiled tomatoes, sausages, or bacon

INGREDIENTS
⅓ cup cold mashed potatoes
⅓ cup milk (breast, formula, cow, or alternative)
⅔ cup all-purpose flour
½ teaspoon baking powder
I medium egg, beaten
sunflower oil, for frying
I cup no-sodium and no-sugar baked beans

8 months

SIMPLE HUMMUS

This delicious alternative to the store-bought dips is made with the calcium-rich sesame seed paste known as tahini, and with chickpeas, a valuable source of iron and the B vitamins. As well as serving it as a dip, you could stir a spoonful into soups and stews.

about 7 child-size servings

finger foods, such as breadsticks, rice cakes, steamed vegetable sticks

INGREDIENTS

¾ cup drained and rinsed
  canned chickpeas
Juice of ½ lemon
½ clove garlic, crushed
1 tablespoon tahini
  (sesame seed paste)
2 tablespoons extra-virgin
  olive oil
2 tablespoons water

1 Put the chickpeas into a food processor or blender with the lemon juice, garlic, tahini, olive oil, and water.

2 Process until pureed—you will have to stir the hummus occasionally during blending to keep the mixture moving. Add extra water if the humous is too thick.

3 Put 1–2 tablespoons into a small bowl and serve with finger foods. Spoon the remainder into an airtight container.

STORAGE TIP

Simple Hummus will keep up to one week stored in the refrigerator in an airtight container.

7-8 months

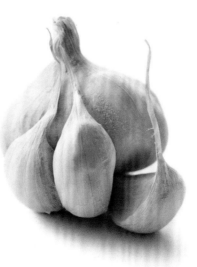

CREAMY GUACAMOLE

Avocados provide useful amounts of protein, carbohydrate, and monounsaturated fat. They also contain the highest concentration of vitamin E of any fruit. The mayonnaise gives this guacamole a creamy consistency, which is more appealing to children, but you could omit the garlic, if preferred.

Put the avocado flesh into a bowl and mash with a fork until smooth. Add the mayonnaise, tomato, garlic, if using, and lemon juice, then mix well until combined.

STORAGE TIP
Creamy Guacamole can be kept in the refrigerator in an airtight container for up to two days.

about 2–4 child-size servings

finger foods, such as breadsticks, rice cakes, steamed vegetable sticks

INGREDIENTS
1 small ripe avocado, pitted and flesh scooped out
1 teaspoon mayonnaise
1 small tomato, peeled, seeded, and finely chopped
½ clove garlic, crushed (optional)
1 teaspoon lemon juice

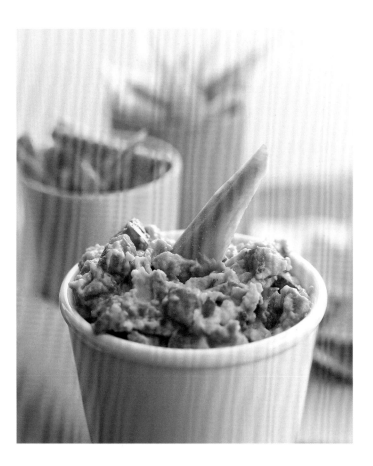

7-8 months

TOMATO & BEAN DIP

This creamy dip makes a quick, nutritious snack. It is delicious spread on different breads or used as a dip with finger foods.

about 10 child-size servings

oatcakes, muffins whole-wheat bread, steamed vegetable sticks

INGREDIENTS

3 vine-ripened tomatoes, quartered and seeded

3 cloves garlic, left whole in their skin

2 tablespoons extra-virgin olive oil

1¼ cups drained and rinsed canned cannellini beans

2 tablespoons lemon juice

1 Preheat the oven to 400°F. Put the tomatoes and garlic with half of the olive oil into a roasting pan. Roast for 15 minutes, until the garlic is soft and the tomatoes tender.

2 Peel the garlic and tomatoes and put into a food processor or blender with the rest of the oil, beans, and lemon juice. Puree the bean mixture until smooth, then store in the refrigerator in an airtight container.

STORAGE TIP

The Tomato & Bean Dip will keep in an airtight container in the refrigerator for up to one week.

7-8 months

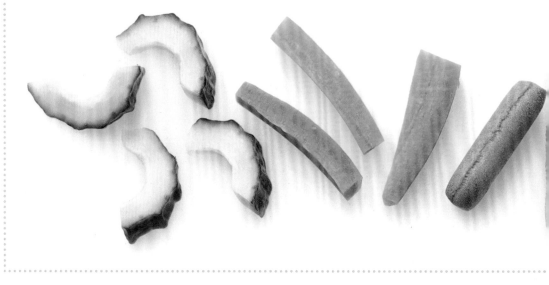

Fresh vegetables, lightly steamed for babies without many teeth, and breadsticks make ideal finger food on their own as well as baby "crudités" for eating with a variety of dips.

EGGPLANT PUREE

Eggplants make a nutritious (rich in the B vitamins and vitamin C) and surprisingly creamy dip.

1 Preheat the oven to 400°F. Put the eggplant in an oiled roasting pan. Roast for 30–35 minutes, or until the flesh is soft when pressed with a finger.

2 Let cool slightly, then cut the eggplant in half lengthwise and scoop out the flesh with a spoon; discard the skin.

3 Put the cooked eggplant into a food processor or blender with the olive oil, garlic, spices, lemon juice, and tahini. Blend to make a smooth and creamy dip.

STORAGE TIP
The Eggplant Dip will keep in an airtight container in the refrigerator for up to one week.

8-9 months

about 4 child-size servings

finger foods, such as breadsticks, rice cakes, steamed vegetables sticks

INGREDIENTS

1 small eggplant
1 tablespoon olive oil, plus extra for greasing
1 clove garlic, chopped
½ teaspoon ground cumin
½ teaspoon ground coriander
Juice of ½ lemon
1 tablespoon tahini (sesame seed paste)

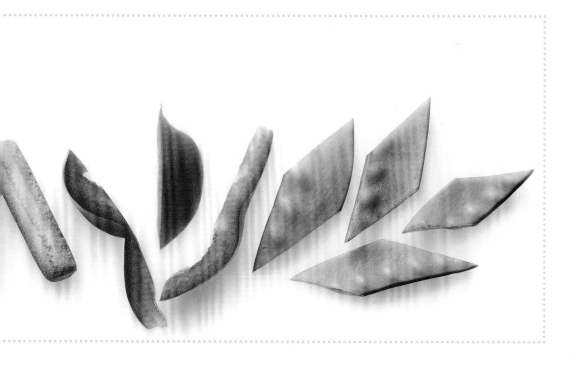

SARDINES ON TOAST

Fresh sardines are incredibly bony so tend not to be popular with children. However, the canned variety make a useful, nutritious alternative and still provide beneficial brain oils. Furthermore, the sardines are mixed with fresh tomato and pesto to dilute any fishiness.

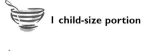 **I child-size portion**

 on their own

INGREDIENTS

I slice whole-wheat bread
2 boned sardines in tomato
   sauce
I heaping teaspoon red pesto
I cherry tomato, seeded and
   chopped

1 Preheat the broiler to medium-high. Line a broiler pan with foil. Mash the sardines and mix with the pesto and tomato.

2 Toast one side of the bread, then turn over and lightly toast the other side. Spoon the sardine mixture on top and broil for 3 minutes, until heated through.

3 Let cool slightly, then cut into strips.

VARIATION

Use other canned fish, such as mackerel or salmon instead of the sardines. All are rich in omega-3 fatty acids.

Pesto contains pine nuts, which are not recommended for babies with a family history of nut allergy.

EGG TOASTS

This makes a fun snack:. Cut out a circle in the center of a slice of bread and replace it with an egg. Add vegetables if serving for lunch.

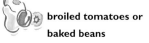 **about I child-size serving**

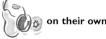 **broiled tomatoes or baked beans**

INGREDIENTS

I slice whole-wheat bread
I egg
butter, for spreading

1 Preheat the broiler to high. Stamp out a circle, about 2 inches in diameter, in the center of the slice of bread, using a pastry cutter.

2 Line the broiler pan with aluminum foil. Toast one side of the bread. Turn the bread over, spread the top with butter, and break the egg into the hole in the center. Broil for about 5 minutes, until both the white and yolk are set.

CINNAMON FRENCH TOAST

This makes a delicious finger food or a brunch dish and also can be served for dessert. The French toast comes with sliced bananas, but you could serve it with any favorite fresh fruit, such as strawberries or sliced pear, to add a nutritional boost.

1 Use a fork to mix together the egg, milk, and cinnamon in a shallow dish. Melt the butter in a nonstick skillet and swirl it around to coat the bottom evenly.

2 Dip both sides of the brioche slice in the egg mixture, then let any excess drip off.

3 Cook for about 2 minutes on each side or until the egg is set and light golden.

1 child-size serving

sliced or mashed banana

INGREDIENTS

1 egg, lightly beaten
1 tablespoon low-fat milk
Pinch of ground cinnamon
Small pat of butter
1 slice bread, brioche,
    or panettone, or 1 small
    fruit roll

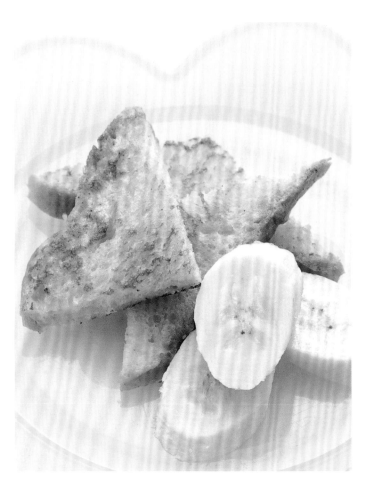

8 months

BREADSTICKS

These breadsticks make an energy-boosting snacks eaten on their own or dipped into hummus or similar alternative. Store in an airtight container for a couple of days, or freeze for future use.

 25 sticks

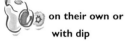 **on their own or with dip**

INGREDIENTS

2 teaspoons olive oil

1¾ cups plus 1 tablespoon white bread flour, plus extra for dusting

1½ teaspoons active dry yeast

½ teaspoon salt (optional)

⅔ cup lukewarm water

1 medium egg, beaten

1 In a large bowl, mix together the flour with the yeast and salt, if using. Add the water and oil, mixing initially with a wooden spoon, and then your hands to make a soft, slightly sticky dough, adding more water or flour if the mixture seems too dry or wet.

2 Dust a work surface with flour and knead the dough for 10 minutes by pushing the dough flat with the palm of your hand, then folding the far edge toward you, giving it a half turn, then repeat the process. Place the dough in a clean bowl, cover with a dish towel, and let it rest somewhere warm and out of a draft for 10 minutes.

3 Preheat the oven to 425°F. Roll out the dough into a thin rectangle, halve the dough horizontally, and cut into ½-inch-wide strips. Roll each piece of dough into a log shape, using both hands, and place on a lightly floured baking sheet. You will need 2 baking sheets, because this dough makes about 25 breadsticks. Cover each sheet with a clean dish towel and set aside for 15 minutes, or until risen.

4 Mix together the beaten egg and milk and brush the mixture lightly over each breadstick. Bake for 15 minutes, until crisp and golden. Transfer to a wire rack to cool.

SEEDY BREADSTICKS

Lightly toast 2 tablespoons of sunflower seeds in a dry skillet. Transfer to a food processor with 1 tablespoon of olive oil and grind to make a coarse paste. Set aside to cool, then mix into the dough mixture in step 1.

CHEESY BREADSTICKS

Roll out the dough into a thin rectangle as in step 3, then sprinkle 1 cup shredded Gruyère cheese over the top. Fold the pastry in half and roll out again to seal the edges. Cut into long ½-inch strips, then cut each strip in half and gently twist. Place on lightly greased baking sheets, brush with the glaze, and bake as above.

8 months

CHEESY PEOPLE

These mini "people-shape" cheese biscuits make a fun snack.

1 Preheat the oven to 425°F and lightly grease two baking sheets. Sift both types of flour and the baking powder into a large bowl.

2 Rub in the butter with your fingertips until the mixture forms coarse bread crumbs. Stir in the cheese and make a hollow in the middle. Pour in the egg and milk and mix initially with a wooden spoon, and then with your hands, to make a soft dough.

3 Turn out the dough oton a lightly floured work surface and gently press into a circle about 1 inch thick. Stamp out the 12 "people," using small gingerbread people cutters. Place on the prepared baking sheets, brush the tops with milk, and bake for 12–15 minutes, until risen and golden. Transfer to a wire rack to cool.

VARIATION

To make cheese biscuits, follow the instructions up to step 3 and after rolling out the dough, use a 2-inch round cutter to stamp out 12 circles. Brush with the egg-and-milk mixture and bake as above.

12 "people"

on their own

INGREDIENTS

1 cup all-purpose flour
1 cup whole-wheat flour
2 teaspoons baking powder
4 tablespoons chilled butter, cubed
3 tablespoons freshly grated Parmesan cheese
1 egg, beaten
½ cup milk, plus extra for glazing

8 months

COUNTRY GARDEN SALAD

It is a good idea to introduce children to salads as early as possible. This is a great one to start with, because it contains a combination of fruit, vegetables, and cheese. They also can eat it with their fingers.

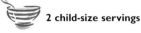 **2 child-size servings**

boiled new potatoes or slice of bread with butter or spread

INGREDIENTS

Dressing

1 tablespoon extra-virgin olive oil

1 teaspoon white wine vinegar

1 teaspoon mayonnaise

Salad

8 cherry tomatoes, halved

4 baby corn, blanched and sliced

8 white or black seedless grapes, halved

4 slices green bell pepper

2 slices American cheese

1 To make the dressing, whisk together the oil, vinegar, and mayonnaise.

2 Put the tomatoes, corn, and grapes and green bell pepper into a bowl. Spoon over the dressing and toss well.

3 Cut the cheese into small pieces and sprinkle them over the top of the salad.

PREPARATION TIP

Encourage your child to eat salad by making it more interesting; the vegetables and cheese can be cut into leaves or flowers, or any shapes you can think of. Feel free to change the ingredients in this salad, depending on likes and dislikes. Carrots, red bell pepper, cucumber, or even toasted nuts and seeds all make delicious additions.

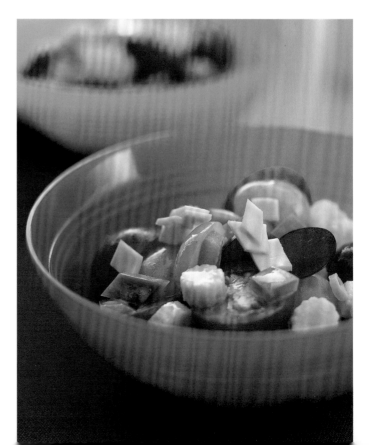

12 months

HALLOUMI & PITA SALAD

This chunky salad is best eaten with the fingers if serving to young children. You could add cubes of Edam or cheddar instead of the halloumi, if preferred, but if sticking to the latter, first give it a rinse to remove any salty residue.

1 Preheat the broiler to medium. Broil the pita bread until light golden and slightly crisp; let cool. Meanwhile, mix together the ingredients for the dressing, if using.

2 Cut the cucumber lengthwise into quarters, then remove the seeds and cut into manageable chunks or sticks. Cut the bell pepper into manageable chunks or sticks.

3 Put the cucumber and bell pepper into a serving bowl, then add the olives, if using. Pour the dressing over the salad and toss until combined.

4 Heat a little oil in a skillet and cook the halloumi until beginning to brown. Let cool to just warm and mix with the rest of the salad. Serve with the pita bread strips.

STORAGE TIP

If not serving this salad at one sitting, store the ingredients individually and keep for up to two days.

1–2 child-size servings

on its own

INGREDIENTS

Salad
1 small pita bread, cut into
   strips
1-inch piece cucumber
¼ small red bel pepper
1 oz halloumi, rinsed, patted
   dry, and cut into cubes
3 pitted black ripe olives,
   halved (optional)

Dressing (optional)
1 tablespoon extra-virgin olive
   oil, plus extra for frying
½ teaspoon white wine
   vinegar

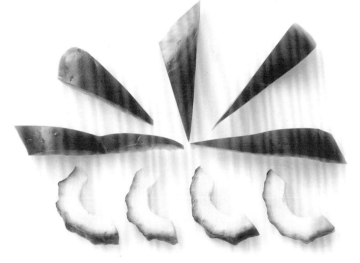

HOMEMADE BAKED BEANS

Canned baked beans often contain excessive amounts of sugar and sodium, but by making your own, you can control what ingredients you use. Beans are nutritious but also high in fiber and, therefore, should not be given to young babies in large quantities, because they may find them difficult to digest.

 2–4 child-size servings

 toast or bread

INGREDIENTS

1 tablespoon olive oil
1 cup drained and rinsed canned low-sugar and low-sodium navy beans
⅔ cup tomato puree
1–2 teaspoons Dijon mustard
1 teaspoon Worcestershire sauce
1 teaspoon maple syrup
1 tablespoon tomato paste

1 Put all the ingredients into a heavy saucepan and mix together thoroughly. Bring to a boil, then reduce the heat and simmer 10 minutes.

2 Cover the pan half and simmer for another 10 minutes, until the beans are tender and the sauce has reduced and thickened.

VARIATION
Serve the beans topped with shredded cheddar cheese.

STORAGE TIP
The baked beans can be kept in the refrigerator in an airtight container for up to two days.

8 months

POTATO & CABBAGE CAKES

Any leftover vegetables can be transformed into these delicious potato cakes—they are a perfect way to encourage children to eat cabbage. They can be mashed or cut into pieces for younger eaters.

1 Cook the potatoes in plenty of boiling salted water for 15 minutes, until tender. Drain well and mash until smooth.

2 Meanwhile, steam the cabbage for 5 minutes, or until tender, then finely chop.

3 Combine the potatoes and cabbage with the mustard, scallions (if using), and egg in a bowl. Mix well with a wooden spoon and let cool.

4 Shape the potato mixture into eight cakes, using floured hands and dusting each cake in flour.

5 Heat enough oil to coat the bottom of a heavy skillet. Cook the cakes, in batches, over medium heat for 3–4 minutes on each side, until golden.

VARIATION
Peas, carrots, green beans, and onion can be used instead of, or as well as, the cabbage. A handful of shredded cheese mixed into the mashed potatoes also tastes great.

8 cakes
I cake will serve an eight month old

broiled tomatoes, beans, or ketchup

INGREDIENTS
6 Yukon gold or russet potatoes, diced
2 cups finely shredded savoy cabbage
I tablespoon Dijon mustard
2 scallions, finely chopped (optional)
I egg, beaten
Flour, for dusting
Vegetable oil, for frying

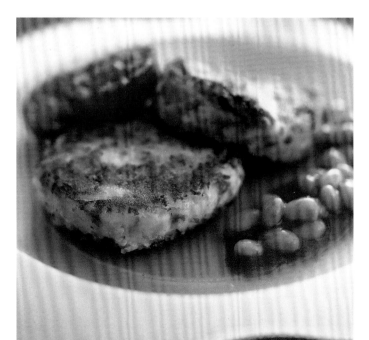

8 months

BAKED POTATOES

Wholesome, nutritious, and easy to prepare, the inside of a baked potato is suitable for babies from six months. The skin can be served as finger food from eight months.

 makes 4

 butter or spread or fillings

INGREDIENTS

4 russet potatoes, washed
Butter or polyunsaturated
   spread

1 Preheat the oven to 400°F. Prick each potato a few times with a fork. Bake for 1–1½ hours, until the skins are crisp and the insides are soft. Cut the potatoes in half.

2 Top the potatoes with butter or spread, or alternatively add one of the fillings suggested opposite.

8 months

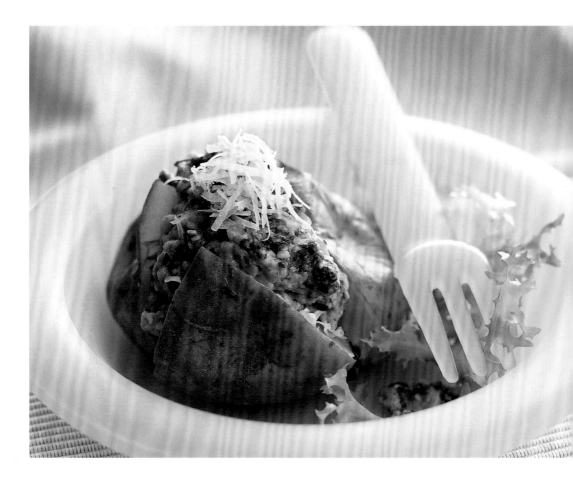

PESTO & AVOCADO FILLING

1 Put the avocado flesh into a bowl and mash with a fork until smooth. Add the mayonnaise, lemon juice, and pesto and mix until combined.

2 Spoon the avocado mixture on top of baked potatoes and sprinkle with Parmesan cheese (if using). If serving to young babies, scoop out the potato and mash with the filling. The skin can be cut into strips and served as finger food if your baby has reached this stage.

Note *Contains pine nuts, which are not recommended for babies with a history of nut allergy within the family.*

INGREDIENTS

I medium avocado, pitted and
flesh scooped out
I tablespoon mayonnaise
I teaspoon lemon juice
I tablespoon green pesto
Freshly grated Parmesan
cheese (optional)

HUMMUS & ROASTED RED PEPPER FILLING

1 While the potatoes are cooking, put the bell pepper onto a baking pan and toss in the oil. Roast for 30-40 minutes, turning occasionally, until tender and the skin is slightly blackened in areas.

2 Put the bell pepper into a plastic bag and let rest for a few minutes; this makes it easier to peel. Remove the skin and cut the bell pepper in half. Scoop out the seeds then finely chop or puree the flesh.

3 Combine the bell pepper with the hummus and olive oil and spoon the mixture over the baked potatoes. If serving to young babies, scoop out the potato and mash with the filling. The skin can be cut into strips and served as finger food if your baby has reached this stage.

INGREDIENTS

I medium red bell pepper,
seeded and sliced
I tablespoon olive oil
¼ cup hummus

CREAM CHEESE & LEEK FILLING

Sauté the leek in the olive oil for 5 minutes, until softened. Remove from the heat and stir in the cream cheese with the chives. Spoon on top of the baked potatoes.

INGREDIENTS

I medium leek, finely chopped
I tablespoon olive oil
¼ cup cream cheese
I tablespoon finely chopped
chives

SESAME POTATO WEDGES

These potato wedges make great finger food. They are healthier than fries, because they retain their nutritious skin and are baked in the oven, which keeps fat levels down. You also can use orange-fleshed sweet potatoes, which are rich in vitamin C and beta-carotene.

2–4 child-size servings

Preheat the oven to 400°F.

low-sugar ketchup, hummus, or dip

2 Toss the potatoes in the oil and put onto a baking pan. Bake for 25 minutes, then remove from the oven. Turn the potatoes, making sure they are thoroughly coated in the oil, and sprinkle with the sesame seeds, if using.

INGREDIENTS

3 russet potatoes, scrubbed and cut into wedges

1 tablespoon olive oil

1 teaspoon sesame seeds (optional)

3 Return the potatoes to the oven for another 15–20 minutes, until tender and golden.

This dish contains seeds—avoid serving to babies if there is a history of nut allergy, asthma, hay fever, or eczema within the immediate family. Please consult your pediatrician.

8-9 months

RICE & VEGETABLE FRITTERS

This recipe is perfect for using up any leftover rice and makes great finger food when cut up. Brown rice is used here because it is a good source of the B vitamins and fiber, but white rice is also suitable.

Mix the rice with the scallions, red bell pepper, garlic, egg, cream, and flour.

2 Heat enough oil to coat the bottom of a heavy skillet. Put 2 tablespoons of the rice mixture per fritter into the hot oil and flatten slightly with the back of a spoon. Cook, in batches, for 3 minutes on each side, until golden, and drain on paper towels

4–8 child-size servings

steamed green beans and broccoli

INGREDIENTS

½ cup long-grain brown rice, cooked and cooled
2 scallions, sliced
½ red bell pepper, diced
1 clove garlic, crushed
1 medium egg, beaten
2 tablespoons heavy cream
2 tablespoons all-purpose flour
Sunflower oil, for frying

7-8 months

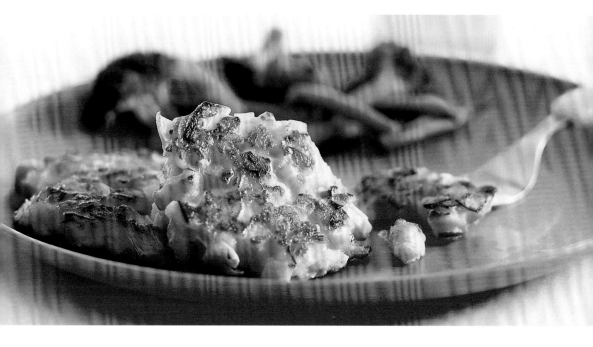

PEA SOUP

Soups are a perfect way of encouraging children to eat vegetables. You could also add less water to make a thicker soup or puree. When your baby is older—12 months or more—you can make the soup with low-sodium broth instead of water.

4 servings
(2 children, 2 adults)

bread sprinkled with shredded cheddar cheese

INGREDIENTS

1 tablespoon vegetable oil
1 leek, finely sliced
1 stick celery, finely chopped
2 Yukon gold or white round
  potatoes, diced
4 cups water
2 cups frozen peas

1 Heat the oil in a large, heavy saucepan. Add the leek and sauté over medium heat for 5 minutes or until softened. Add the celery and potato and cook for another 5 minutes.

2 Pour the water over the vegetables and bring to a boil. Cover, reduce the heat, and simmer the soup for 15 minutes. Add the peas and cook for another 5 minutes or until the potato is tender.

3 Using a handheld blender or food processor, blend the soup until smooth. Reheat the soup, if necessary, before serving. For the adult servings, season to taste with salt and black pepper.

STORING TIP

Soups freeze well and will keep for up to three months. You could freeze the Pea Soup in convenient child-size portions.

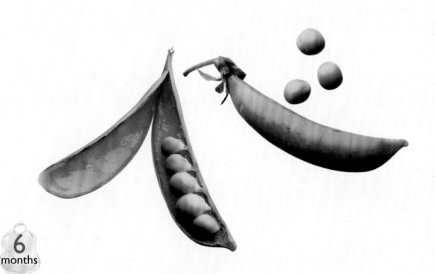

6 months

MISO NOODLE SOUP

This soup is very quick to make because it has a base of instant miso soup. Miso is made from fermented soybeans and is rich in minerals, particularly iron and calcium.

1 Steam the green beans and carrot until tender.

2 Meanwhile, cook the noodles in plenty of boiling water following the package directions. Add the spinach 2 minutes before the end of the cooking time. Drain the noodles and spinach and cut into manageable-size pieces.

3 Make the miso soup, following the package directions. Put the noodles, carrots, and beans into a serving bowl; chop them first if suitable for your baby. Pour the miso soup over the top. Stir in the soy sauce, if using.

4 Let the soup cool to the right temperature, then serve garnished with the scallion and sesame seeds (if using).

2 child-size servings

to make a more substantial soup, add ground cubes of marinated tofu or strips of cooked chicken.

INGREDIENTS

6 fine green beans, finely chopped
I small carrot, finely chopped
I envelope instant miso soup powder
2 oz egg or rice noodles
Handful of fresh baby spinach leaves, shredded
I teaspoon reduced-sodium soy sauce (optional)
I scallion, finely shredded and sesame seeds, to garnish (optional)

Note The soup contains seeds and soy, both of which have been linked to allergies. Avoid if there is any history of allergies in the family.

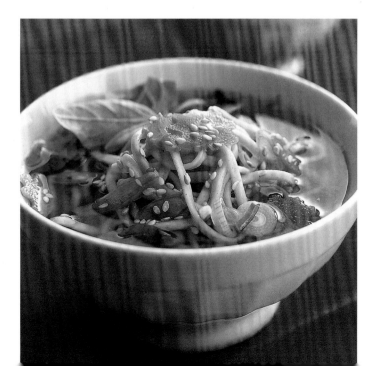

TOMATO & LENTIL SOUP

Tomato soup is a national favorite but store-bought versions contain a surprising amount of fat and sugar. This nutritious homemade version features the added health benefit of lentils and doesn't take an age to make. With babies older than 12 months, you can make the soup with low-sodium broth and add a dash of black pepper.

**4 servings
(2 children, 2 adults)**

**bread sprinkled with
shredded cheddar cheese**

INGREDIENTS

¼ cup split red lentils, rinsed
1 tablespoon olive oil
1 onion, chopped
1 carrot, finely chopped
1 stick celery, finely chopped
2 cups tomato puree
2 cups water
1 bay leaf
3 tablespoons milk (optional)

1 Put the lentils into a saucepan, cover with water, and bring to a boil. Reduce the heat and simmer, half-covered, for 15 minutes or until just tender. Remove any scum that rises to the surface, using a spoon. Drain the lentils well and set aside.

2 Heat the oil in a large, heavy saucepan. Add the onion, cover the pan, and sauté for 8 minutes, until softened and transparent. Add the carrot and celery, cover, and cook for another 3 minutes, stirring occasionally to prevent the vegetables from sticking to the bottom of the pan.

3 Add the tomato puree, water, lentils, and bay leaf. Bring to a boil. Reduce the heat and simmer, half-covered, for 30 minutes, until the lentils and vegetables are tender and the soup has thickened.

4 Carefully pour the soup into a blender or use a handheld blender to puree the soup until smooth. Return to the pan and stir in the milk, if using. Reheat, if necessary, and serve.

STORAGE TIP
Tomato & Lentil Soup can be kept for up to three months in the freezer. Try freezing the soup in convenient-size portions.

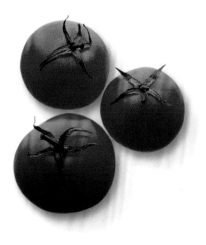

6 months

MUFFIN PIZZAS

Children love pizzas and they make great finger food. English muffins are used as the crust for these simple pizzas, but you could also use pita bread or rolls. Why not add your favorite toppings, too.

1 Preheat the broiler to medium. Mix together the tomato puree (if using canned tomatoes, mash them with a fork until fairly smooth), pesto or paste, olive oil, and oregano, if using, to create a sauce.

2 Cover the top of each muffin half with half of the tomato sauce.

3 Top with a slice of mozzarella, then broil for 8–10 minutes, or until the cheese has melted and is slightly golden. Cut each muffin half into quarters to make them more manageable to eat and let cool to the right temperature.

1–2 child-size servings

vegetable fingers

INGREDIENTS

2 tablespoons tomato puree or canned diced tomatoes
1 teaspoon tomato pesto or tomato paste
½ teaspoon olive oil
Pinch of dried oregano (optional)
1 English muffin, halved horizontally
2 slices mozzarella, drained, patted dry

Note *Tomato pesto contains pine nuts, which are not recommended for babies with a family history of nut allergy.*

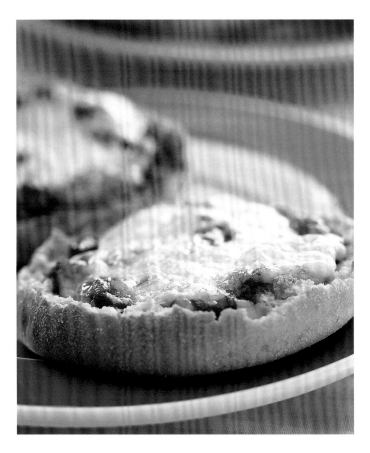

8 months

MINI QUICHES

These baby-size pies are just the right size for small hands to handle. Here, puff pastry is used but you could use flaky pastry, if preferred.

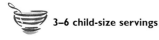

3–6 child-size servings

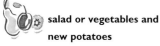

salad or vegetables and new potatoes

INGREDIENTS

Butter, for greasing
1 sheet ready-to-bake puff
   pastry, defrosted if frozen
3 large eggs, beaten
½ cup milk
½ cup shredded sharp
   cheddar cheese
1 medium tomato, sliced

1 Preheat the oven to 400°F. Grease a deep six-cup muffin pan. Roll out the puff pastry until it is thin and press it into the six muffin cups. Trim the tops and chill the pastry for 30 minutes.

2 Combine the beaten eggs, milk, and cheese, reserving a little cheese for sprinkling. Pour the mixture into the muffin pan and top each quiche with a slice of tomato, then sprinkle with the reserved cheese.

3 Bake for 20–25 minutes, until risen and golden. Let cool slightly before removing the quiches from the pan.

12 months

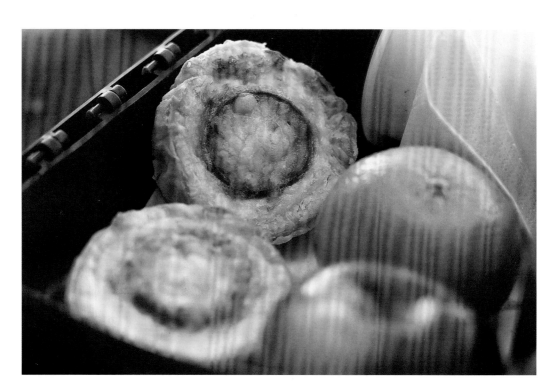

BABY FALAFEL BURGERS

These nutritious burgers are made from chickpeas, which are a good source of iron, zinc, folate, and vitamin E.

1 Put the chickpeas, scallions, garlic, cumin, and coriander into a food processor and blend. Add the egg and blend again until the mixture forms a coarse paste. Then place the mixture in the refrigerator for 1 hour.

2 Remove the chickpea paste from the refrigerator and, with floured hands, form into six patties, about 2½ inches in diameter. Roll each one in flour until lightly coated.

3 Heat enough oil to cover the bottom of a large skillet. Cook the piatties (in batches and adding more oil, if necessary) for 6 minutes, turning once, until golden.

4 Serve each patty in a mini bread roll with slices of cucumber and tomato, with a dollop of hummus, mayonnaise, or ketchup. Or, to serve as finger food, cut the patty and roll into pieces and serve the hummus, mayonnaise, or ketchup on the side as a dip.

STORAGE TIP
The Baby Falafel Burgers can be frozen cooked or uncooked. Store them with a sheet of baking paper between each patty and then stacked into a pile. Put them in a freezer bag for future use.

6 burgers
1 burger will serve an eight month old
cucumber and tomato slices and hummus, mayonnaise, or low-sugar ketchup

INGREDIENTS

1 (15-oz) can chickpeas, drained and rinsed
3 scallions, chopped
2 cloves garlic, crushed
1 teaspoon ground cumin
1 teaspoon ground coriander
1 egg, beaten
Flour, for dusting
Vegetable oil, for frying
6 mini bread rolls or pita breads

8-9 months

MOZZARELLA TORTILLA PACKAGE

A great alternative to the usual cheese sandwich, this crispy, warm tortilla is filled with melted mozzarella, pesto, and tomato—any fillings can be used, depending on what you have on hand. Serve with slices of carrot and cucumber.

1–2 child-size servings

slices of carrot and cucumber

INGREDIENTS

2 slices mozzarella
1 soft tortilla
2 slices tomato
1 teaspoon pesto
1 teaspoon olive oil

1 Place the mozzarella in the center of the tortilla. Top with the slices of tomato and the pesto. Fold in the sides of the tortilla to make a square package.

2 Heat the oil in a heavy skillet with a lid. Place the package seam side down in the skillet. Cover the pan and cook over low heat for about 3 minutes, turning once, until golden. Halve diagonally and serve.

BABY BREADS

Tempt your baby with an out-of-the ordinary sandwich. All babies enjoy bread cut into shapes or into strips, then rolled around a filling, but you also can make use of the variety of mini breads and rolls available. Pita breads and bagels are available in small sizes, as are many shaped rolls. They also can be bought as whole-wheat versions. Croissants, too, can be found in smaller sizes and make delicious and easy-to-hold sandwich bases.

Note Pesto contains pine nuts, which are not recommended for babies with a family history of nut allergy.

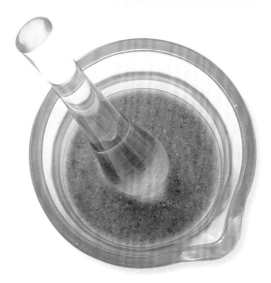

12 months

EGG ROLLS

This speedy dish of scrambled egg in a tortilla is a good source of iron, the B vitamins, and phosphorus. If your baby has difficulty holding the roll, serve the egg separately and cut the tortilla into strips; this would be suitable for babies from seven to eight months..

1 Heat the butter and oil in a heavy saucepan, add the bell pepper and scallion, and sauté for 5 minutes, until softened.

2 Beat together the eggs and milk and pour the mixture into the pan. Using a wooden spoon, stir constantly, to make sure the egg doesn't stick. Continue to cook the egg, stirring, for about 4 minutes, until there is no trace of runniness.

3 Remove from the heat—the egg will keep warm due to the heat from the pan. Warm the tortillas in an oven or a dry skillet, then spoon the scrambled egg on top and roll up. Cut in half horizontally and serve.

2–4 child-size servings

on their own

INGREDIENTS

Pat of unsalted butter
1 teaspoon olive oil
¼ red bell pepper, seeded and diced
1 scallion, finely chopped
4 eggs, lightly beaten
2 tablespoons milk
2 soft tortillas

TUNA TORTILLA MELT

Tuna is one of the oily fish family providing omega-3 fats, essential for brain development and function. Although canned tuna is lower in these beneficial oils than fresh tuna, it still provides useful amounts as well as valuable protein. Soft, floury tortillas are perfect for filling with all kinds of healthy goodies.

 1–2 child-size servings

steamed carrots and corn kernels

INGREDIENTS

3½ oz canned tuna in spring water or olive oil, drained

1 large soft tortilla

¼ cup shredded sharp cheddar cheese

1 small tomato, seeded and finely chopped

1 Mash the drained tuna with a fork and arrange it in the center of the tortilla. Top with the cheddar cheese and sliced tomato.

2 Fold in the edges of the tortilla to encase the filling. Heat a dry, nonstick skillet over medium heat. Place the tortilla, seam side down, in the pan and cook for 3–5 minutes, until warmed through and golden. Cut in half diagonally and serve.

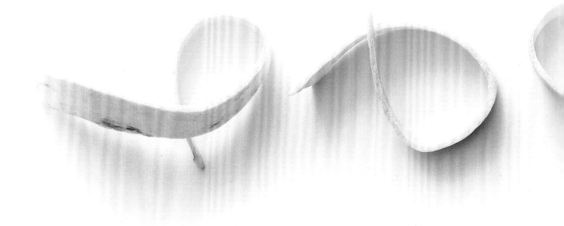

 12 months

QUICK & EASY SAUSAGE ROLLS

Use the best sausages that you can find and you won't be filling your children with unwanted additives. And if you're using store-bought bottled sauces to serve, look for the "no-added sugar and sodium" varieties. If your baby can't handle the roll, serve the sausages ground or finely chopped and separate from the tortilla strips, which can be served separately.

1 Preheat the broiler to medium-high. Line a broiler pan with aluminum foil and arrange the sausages on top. Broil the sausages until cooked through and golden.

2 Place the tortilla strips in a dry skillet and heat until warmed through. Spread a little of the topping of your choice over the each strip and top with a sausage. Roll up each strip to encase the sausage.

1–2 child-size servings

mayonnaise, ketchup, guacamole, or hummus

INGREDIENTS

4 good-quality cocktail pork sausages or vegetarian alternative

1 small soft flour tortilla, cut into four strips

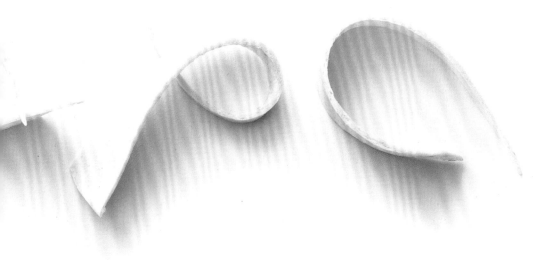

MACARONI & CHEESE WITH LEEKS

A family favorite for all ages, macaroni and cheese is great comfort food that provides calcium for strong teeth and bones. Puree, grind, or finely chop, depending on the age of your baby.

**4 servings
(2 children, 2 adults)**

steamed vegetables

INGREDIENTS

4 oz macaroni

4 tablespoons butter

3 leeks, trimmed and chopped

¼ cup all-purpose flour

3 cups milk (breast, formula, cow, or alternative)

1 heaping teaspoon dry English mustard

2 tablespoons crème fraîche or plain Greek yogurt

½ cup finely grated Parmesan cheese

1 cup shredded cheddar cheese

1 Cook the macaroni in a large saucepan of boiling water following the package directions.

2 Melt the butter in a medium, heavy saucepan, then add the leeks and sauté for 4 minutes, until softened.

3 Stir in the flour and cook for 1 minute, stirring continuously. Gradually add the milk, stirring all the time with a whisk to avoid any lumps. When all of the milk has been added, stir in the mustard. Preheat the broiler to high.

4 Bring the white sauce to a boil, then reduce the heat and simmer for 5 minutes, stirring frequently. Stir in the crème fraiche or yogurt, half of the Parmesan, and two-thirds of the cheddar and heat through until the cheese has melted.

5 Drain the pasta, reserving 3 tablespoons of the cooking water. Return the pasta and water to the pan and pour in the cheese sauce. Turn until the pasta is coated in the sauce, then transfer to a warm ovenproof dish.

6 Sprinkle the remaining Parmesan and cheddar over the top and broil for 6–8 minutes, until the top is golden.

VARIATION

In addition to the leeks, you could add steamed broccoli or peas and top the macaroni with slices of tomato.

STORAGE TIP

Macaroni & Cheese with Leeks will keep stored in the refrigerator in an airtight container for up to three days or can be frozen for up to three months.

6 months

POTATO, PEA & PESTO PASTA

It's a good idea to familiarize babies and young children with strong flavors, and pesto is ideal for this. You could use a prepared alternative, if preferred. Peas are definitely a favorite with most children.

1 First make the pesto. Put the basil, garlic, and pine nuts into a food processor and process until finely chopped. Gradually add the olive oil, then the Parmesan and blend to a course puree. Season to taste.

2 Cook the pasta in plenty of boiling salted water following the package directions, until just tender. Add the peas 2 minutes before the end of the cooking time. Drain, reserving 3 tablespoons of the cooking water, and return the pasta and peas to the saucepan.

3 Meanwhile, boil the potatoes for 10 minutes, or until tender. Drain and let cool slightly before cutting into bite-size pieces.

4 Add the potatoes to the peas and pasta, and stir in half of the pesto. Add a little extra olive oil if the sauce appears dry. Stir well, but gently, until the peas and pasta are thoroughly coated, and then heat through.

5 Serve sprinkled with Parmesan cheese then puree, grind, or chop as required; you may need to add a little extra water.

STORAGE TIP

Any remaining pesto can be stored in an airtight jar in the refrigerator for up to a week.

4 servings
(2 children, 2 adults)

steamed broccoli

INGREDIENTS

12 oz pasta wheels or shape
  of your choice
½ cup frozen peas
1 lb baby new potatoes,
  scrubbed and halved
Olive oil, for drizzling
Freshly grated Parmesan,
  to serve

Pesto

6 cups fresh basil leaves
  (stems removed)
1 clove garlic, crushed
3 tablespoons pine nuts
⅓ cup olive oil
⅓ cup freshly grated
  Parmesan cheese

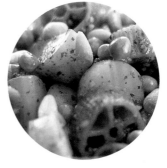

Note *Pesto contains pine nuts—avoid serving to babies if there is a history of nut allergy, asthma, hay fever, or eczema within the immediate family. Please consult your pediatrician.*

SPAGHETTI WITH ROASTED BUTTERNUT SQUASH

Butternut squash has a delicious sweetness that is enhanced when roasted. This simple pasta dish is a favorite with babies and older children alike. Puree, mash, or finely chop, depending on the age of your baby; the pine nuts can be finely chopped or ground.

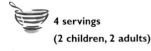

**4 servings
(2 children, 2 adults)**

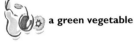

a green vegetable

INGREDIENTS

1 small butternut squash, peeled, seeded, and cubed
3 tablespoons olive oil
2 sprigs fresh rosemary (optional)
12 oz spaghetti
1 large clove garlic, finely chopped
1 tablespoon freshly chopped parsley (optional)
⅓ cup pine nuts, toasted and finely chopped (optional)
Freshly grated Parmesan cheese, to serve

1 Preheat the oven to 400°F. Toss the butternut squash in half of the olive oil and arrange on a baking pan; place the rosemary, if using, on top. Roast the squash for 25 minutes, turning occasionally, until tender. Remove from the oven and set aside.

2 Meanwhile, cook the spaghetti in plenty of boiling water following the package directions. Drain, reserving 2 tablespoons of the cooking water, and return the pasta and water to the pan.

3 Heat the remaining olive oil in a skillet and sauté the garlic for 1 minute, until softened but not browned. Add the garlic and the oil to the pasta with the squash and parsley, if using. Stir well until combined and heat through.

4 Serve the pasta with a sprinkling of the toasted pine nuts, if desired, and Parmesan, if using.

STORAGE TIP

Spaghetti with Roasted Butternut Squash will keep in the refrigerator in an airtight container for up to two days or you can freeze it for up to three months.

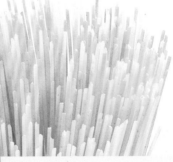

6 months

Note Contains pine nuts—avoid serving to babies if there is a history of nut allergy, asthma, hay fever, or eczema within the immediate family. Please consult your pediatrician.

CREAMY BROCCOLI PASTA CASSEROLE

Broccoli contains many nutrients, including calcium, iron, zinc, the B vitamins, and vitamin C. It can be a real struggle to get children to eat their greens, but cutting them small and immersing them in a creamy cheese sauce seems to make them more palatable.

1 Cook the pasta in plenty of boiling, salted water according to the package directions. Add the broccoli and cauliflower to the pasta 5 minutes before the end of the cooking time. Drain the pasta and vegetables well and transfer to a large bowl.

2 Meanwhile, make the cheese sauce. Melt the butter in a heavy saucepan. Stir in the flour and cook for about 2 minutes, stirring continuously, or until the mixture forms a thick brown paste. Remove from the heat and gradually add the warm milk a little at a time, whisking well with a wire whisk after each addition. Continue to add the milk until the cheese sauce is smooth and creamy.

3 Return the cheese sauce to the heat and add the mustard, if using, and cream cheese. Cook for about 10 minutes, until the sauce has thickened. Mix in the cheddar cheese, reserving some to sprinkle over the top of the casserole, and stir well until it has melted. Pour the sauce over the pasta and vegetables in the bowl and mix gently until combined.

4 Preheat the broiler to high. Transfer the pasta and vegetables to an ovenproof dish and sprinkle with more cheddar cheese and the bread crumbs. Broil for 5–10 minutes, until the cheese is bubbling and the bread crumbs are golden brown. Puree, mash, or finely chop, depending on the age of your child.

VARIATION
Instead of broccoli and cauliflower, other vegetables, such as peas, carrots, leeks, and green beans, can be used.

**4 servings
(2 children, 2 adults)**

steamed carrots

INGREDIENTS
4 oz pasta spirals
2½ cups small broccoli florets
⅔ cup small cauliflower florets
2 tablespoons butter
3 tablespoons all-purpose flour
3 cups milk, warmed
1 tablespoon Dijon mustard (optional)
2 tablespoons cream cheese
1 cup shredded sharp cheddar cheese, plus extra for sprinkling
2 tablespoons fresh bread crumbs

6 months

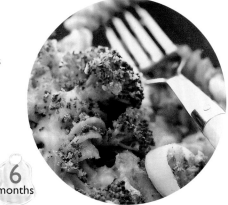

BABY VEGETABLE RISOTTO

Risotto is simple to make but does require stirring time, but can be therapeutic after a hectic day. Puree or mash, depending on your baby's age. Once your baby is 12 months, you can prepare the risotto with low-sodium vegetable broth instead of water.

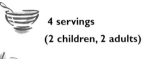

4 servings
(2 children, 2 adults)

steamed carrots

INGREDIENTS

2 tablespoons olive oil
1½ tablespoons butter
4 baby leeks, sliced
4 baby zucchini, sliced
1 teaspoon dried oregano
1⅓ cups risotto rice
4 cups water
⅓ cup peas
1 cup grated Parmesan cheese

1 Heat the oil and butter in a large, heavy saucepan. Add the leeks and zucchini and sauté for 5 minutes or until tender. Add the oregano and rice and cook for 2 minutes, stirring continuously, until the rice is glossy and slightly translucent.

2 Add the water, a ladleful at a time, stirring continuously. Wait for the water to be absorbed before adding another ladleful. Continue in this way until the rice is tender and creamy but still retains a little bite—it should take about 25 minutes.

3 Add the peas, the last spoonful of water, and three-quarters of the Parmesan cheese and stir well. Sprinkle with the remaining Parmesan just before serving.

6 months

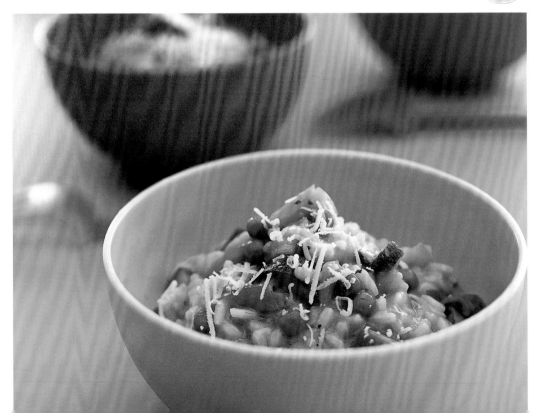

PESTO & PEA RISOTTO

Pesto is a popular sauce served with pasta, but it works equally well stirred into rice or spooned over baked potatoes. To make your own, see the recipe on page 95. Risotto is a great dish for babies and one that is relatively easy for them to serve themselves. Once your baby is 12 months, you can use low-sodium vegetable broth instead of water.

1 Heat the water in a saucepan and add half of the peas. When cooked, scoop out the peas, using a slotted spoon, and transfer to a blender with a ladleful of water. Blend the peas until pureed and set aside.

2 Heat the oil and butter in a large, heavy saucepan and sauté the onions over low heat for 10 minutes, until softened. Add the garlic and sauté for another minute.

3 Pour in the rice and stir until it is coated in the onion mixture. Add a ladleful of water and simmer, stirring, until the liquid is absorbed. Continue to add water, a ladleful at a time, until the liquid is almost fully absorbed and the rice is tender and creamy in texture; this will take 20–25 minutes.

4 Stir in the pea puree, pesto, and half of the Parmesan and heat though. Season with black pepper, if using, and serve sprinkled with the remaining Parmesan.

STORAGE TIP

Pesto & Pea Risotto will keep stored in the refrigerator in an airtight container for up to two days or can be frozen for up to three months. Reheat thoroughly—you may need to add a little water— before serving.

Note *Pesto contains pine nuts; avoid serving to babies if there is a history of nut allergy, asthma, hay fever, or eczema within the immediate family. Please consult your pediatrician.*

4 servings

(2 children, 2 adults)

broiled tomatoes

INGREDIENTS

4 cups water
1⅔ cups frozen pea
1 tablespoon olive oil
1¾ tablespoons butter
2 onions, finely chopped
2 large cloves garlic, finely
   chopped
1⅓ cups risotto rice
⅓ cup pesto
½ cup finely grated
   Parmesan cheese
Freshly ground black pepper
   (optional)

MEXICAN RICE

This nutritionally balanced, lightly spiced meal is delicious topped with shredded cheddar cheese or a spoonful of guacamole or hummus. Brown rice is more nutritious than white, but it is also higher in fiber, so you may prefer to substitute white rice here.

**4 servings
(2 children, 2 adults)**

**tortilla chips; no-sodium
variety is preferred**

INGREDIENTS

1 cup brown rice, rinsed
½ low-sodium vegetable
   bouillon cube (optional)
½ cup sliced fine green beans
1 large carrot, finely diced
1 teaspoon ground cumin
   (optional)
½ teaspoon mild curry
   powder (optional)
¾ cup canned kidney beans,
   drained and rinsed
6 medium tomatoes, halved
   and seeded
1 onion, sliced
2 cloves garlic, unpeeled
1 tablespoon olive oil
shredded cheddar cheese,
   to serve

1 Preheat the oven to 350°F. Put the rice into a saucepan and cover with water (the water level should be about ¾ inch above the rice). Add the bouillon cube, if using, then bring to a boil. Reduce the heat, cover, and simmer for 30 minutes, or until the rice is tender.

2 Add the green beans, carrot, spices (if using), and kidney beans and stir thoroughly. Cook for another 5–10 minutes, or until all of the water has been absorbed. Remove from the heat and let stand, covered, for 5 minutes.

3 Meanwhile, put the tomatoes, onion, and garlic into a baking dish and toss them in the oil until thoroughly coated. Roast for 20 minutes, or until the tomatoes are tender. Transfer to a blender or food processor and puree.

4 Add the tomato puree to the rice-and-bean mixture and stir until mixture is thoroughly coated. Sprinkle with shredded cheddar cheese and serve.

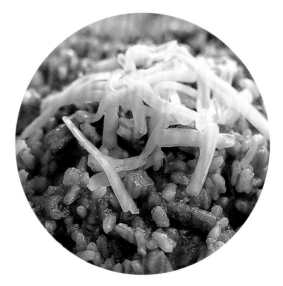

12 months

VEGETABLE STICKS

These vegetarian alternatives to fish sticks are dipped in cornmeal, which gives them a delicious golden crispy coating, but you could use fresh bread crumbs instead. The sticks are a useful way of disguising vegetables if your child dislikes anything remotely green. Finely chopped broccoli, grated cabbage, finely chopped carrots, or green beans can also be used.

1 Cook the potatoes chunks in plenty of boiling water for 10–15 minutes, until tender. Add the peas 2 minutes before the end of the cooking time. Drain the vegetables and let cool.

2 While the potatoes and peas are cooking, steam the leeks for 5–8 minutes, until tender. Squeeze the leeks to get rid of any excess water and combine with the potatoes and peas. Mash well. Let cool completely. When the mixture is cool, stir in the cheese.

3 Sprinkle the cornmeal on a plate until covered. Take 2 heaping tablespoons of the mashed potatos and, using your hands, form them into a log-shape stick. Roll each stick in the cornmeal and turn until completely coated. Continue until you have used all of the potato mixture.

4 Heat enough oil to cover the bottom of a heavy skillet. Cook the sticks, in batches, for 3 minutes on each side, or until heated through and golden.

2–4 child-size servings

steamed peas and carrots

INGREDIENTS

4 Yukon gold or russet
potatoes, cut into chunks
⅓ cup frozen peas
1 leek, finely chopped
½ cup drained, canned
   no-sugar and no-sodium
   corn kernels,
½ cup shredded cheddar
   cheese
Cornmeal, for coating
Vegetable oil, for
   frying

**8
months**

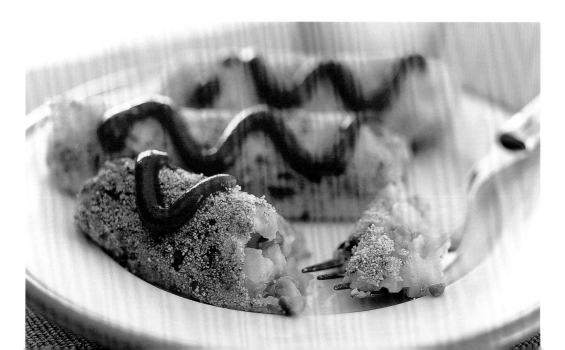

SWEET POTATO CASSEROLE

This delicious casserole is simple comfort food and just the thing for a cold winter's night. It is an attractive, colorful dish, made with vibrant orange layers of sweet potatoes and a bright green layer of leeks, spinach, and peas. Puree, mash, or grind, depending on the age of your baby.

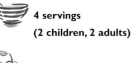

**4 servings
(2 children, 2 adults)**

**low-sugar and low-
sodium baked beans**

INGREDIENTS

5 Yukon gold or russet
  potatoes, peeled and diced
2 sweet potatoes, peeled and
  diced (use the orange-flesh
  variety)
2 tablespoons olive oil
1 large leek, finely chopped
1 tablespoon dried oregano
  or thyme
3 cups trimmed and chopped
  spinach (optional)
¾ cup frozen peas
4 tablespoons unsalted butter,
  plus extra for greasing
⅔ cup milk, warmed
2 tablespoons heavy cream
  (optional)
1 tablespoon Dijon mustard
¾ cup shredded
  cheddar cheese

1 Preheat the oven to 400°F. Cook the potatoes and sweet potatoes in plenty of boiling salted water for 15–20 minutes, or until tender.

2 Meanwhile, heat the oil in a heavy skillet and sauté the leek for 5 minutes, until softened. Add the oregano or thyme and the spinach (if using), then cook for another 3 minutes. Stir in the peas and remove from the heat.

3 Drain the potatoes well and add the butter, warmed milk, cream (if using), and mustard. Mash the potatoes well until smooth and creamy. Butter an ovenproof dish and spoon half of the mashed potatoes into the dish. Smooth with the back of a spoon and top with the leek mixture. Spoon the rest of the mashed potatoes over the top of the leeks and sprinkle with the cheddar cheese. Bake the casserole for 20 minutes, until golden.

6 months

ROASTED VEGETABLE TART

If it's a struggle to get your children to eat vegetables, this delicious tart is the answer, because the roasted vegetables are pureed until they are smooth and creamy. It makes a delicious alternative to a Sunday roast.

1 Preheat the oven to 400°F. Put the squash, garlic, onions, and red pepper into a roasting dish. Toss in the oil and top with the fresh herbs, then roast for 20 minutes.

2 Remove from the oven and add the tomatoes. Turn the vegetables in the oil and return to the oven for another 15 minutes, or until tender.

3 Remove the fresh herbs and garlic and discard. Put the tomatoes into a food processor, along with the rest of the vegetables. Blend until smooth, then let the mixture cool.

4 Lay the sheet of puff pastry on a baking sheet. Brush the edge of the pastry with egg, then fold over to make a lip and seal with your fingers. Spoon the roasted vegetable mixture over the pastry, leaving a gap around the edge.

5 Sprinkle with the cheese. Brush the folded edge of the pastry with egg and bake for 15 minutes, until the pastry has risen and is golden.

VARIATION

Serve the vegetable mixture combined with rice or pasta (omitting the pastry) and sprinkle with a little shredded cheddar cheese.

8 months

**4 servings
(2 children, 2 adult)**

roasted potatoes and steamed vegetables

INGREDIENTS

½ butternut squash, peeled, seeded, and cubed
2 cloves garlic
2 red onions, quartered
1 red bell pepper, cored, seeded, and sliced
3 tablespoons olive oil
2 sprigs fresh rosemary
3 sprigs fresh basil
3 tomatoes, halved and seeded
1 sheet ready-to-bake puff pastry, defrosted, if necessary
1 egg, beaten, to glaze
½ cup shredded cheddar cheese

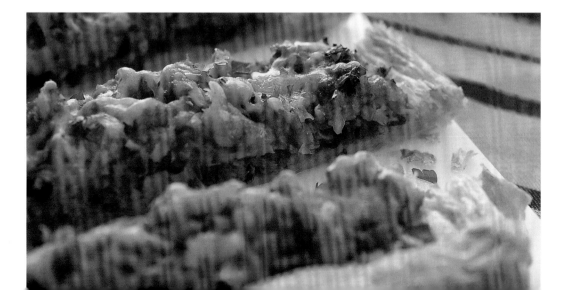

INDIAN LENTIL SOUP

Children often like stronger flavors than adults give them credit for, and it's a good idea to familiarize infants with new tastes. The lentil is much underrated but this low-fat, protein-rich legume provides iron, folic acid, and zinc as well as fiber, and its mild flavor combines well with spices. Adults may like to add a chopped fresh chile.

**4 servings
(2 children, 2 adults)**

basmati or other long-grain rice, naan, or a similar Indian flatbread and a green vegetable

INGREDIENTS

2 tablespoons sunflower oil
1 large onion, chopped
2 large cloves garlic, crushed
4 cardamom pods, halved
   lengthwise
2 bay leaves
2 carrots, shredded
2 tablespoons grated
   fresh ginger
2 teaspoon ground coriander
1 cup red split lentils
2 cups water
1 cup reduced-fat
   coconut milk
1 cup tomato puree or
   canned diced tomatoes
2 teaspoons garam masala
Juice of 1 lime
¼ cup chopped fresh cilantro
   (optional)

1 Heat 1 tablespoon of the oil in a large, heavy saucepan and sauté the onion for 10 minutes, or until softened, stirring frequently. Add the garlic and sauté for another 30 seconds, stirring, followed by the cardamom, bay leaves, carrots, ginger, and ground coriander.

2 After 1 minute, add the lentils, water, coconut milk, and tomato puree to the pan, stir, and bring to a boil, then reduce the heat and simmer, covered, for 20 minutes. Stir in the garam masala and lime juice and cook, covered, for another 20 minutes, stirring occasionally.

3 When the lentils are tender, remove the pan from the heat and remove the whole spices, then puree with a handheld blender until smooth. Stir in the chopped cilantro, if using.

STORAGE TIP

Indian Lentil Soup will keep stored in the refrigerator in an airtight container for up to five days or can be frozen for up to three months.

12 months

TOMATO & TUNA GNOCCHI

Canned tuna is a valuable source of protein and brain-boosting omega-3 essential fatty acids, albeit in lower quantities than fresh fish. Gnocchi are Italian potato dumplings and are the ultimate comfort food. This meal is so quick to prepare and delicious, it's sure to become a family favorite.

1 Heat the oil in a saucepan over medium heat and sauté the garlic for about 30 seconds. Stir in the oregano, then the diced tomatoes.

2 Bring the sauce to a boil, then reduce the heat to low. Half-cover the pan with a lid and simmer for about 10 minutes, or until the sauce has reduced and thickened slightly.

3 Meanwhile, bring a saucepan of water to a boil. Add the gnocchi and return the water to a boil, then stir gently and cook for 1 minute, or according to the package directions; drain.

4 Stir the tuna into the tomato sauce. Half-cover the pan with a lid and heat through gently for 2 minutes, stirring the sauce occasionally.

5 Return the gnocchi to the saucepan and pour in enough tuna sauce to coat, turning it until covered. To serve to babies of six months, puree the dish and add a little extra water.

STORAGE TIP

Homemade tomato sauce (without tuna) is a useful standby and can be kept in the refrigerator in an airtight container for up to one week or frozen for up to three months. The complete dish will keep chilled for up to two days and can be reheated before serving.

4 servings
(2 children, 2 adults)

a salad or green vegetable

INGREDIENTS

1 teaspoon olive oil
2 cloves garlic, finely chopped
1 teaspoon dried oregano (optional)
1 (14½-oz) can diced tomatoes or 1⅔ cups tomato puree or sauce
1 tablespoon tomato puree
1 (5-oz) can tuna in olive oil, drained
Packaged gnocchi (12–20 for children, depending on ages, plus extra for adults)

6 months

TUNA & LEEK FRITTATA

A protein-rich, nutritious dish, this Spanish-style tortilla can be eaten hot or cold and makes a great family dish as well as finger food. If your baby is unable to handle finger food, grind it or finely chop.

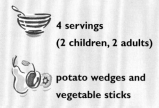

**4 servings
(2 children, 2 adults)**

**potato wedges and
vegetable sticks**

INGREDIENTS

1 tablespoon olive oil
small pat of butter
1 large leek, finely sliced
1 (5-oz) can tuna in olive oil
   or spring water, drained
6 eggs, beaten

1 Heat the oil and butter in a medium, ovenproof skillet, then sauté the leek for 5–7 minutes, or until softened. Stir in the tuna, making sure that there is an even distribution of leek and tuna and that some chunks of tuna remain.

2 Preheat the broiler to medium-high. Pour the eggs evenly over the tuna-and-leek mixture. Cook over medium heat for 5 minutes, or until the eggs are just set and the bottom of the frittata is golden brown.

3 Place the pan under the broiler and cook the top of the frittata for 3 minutes or until set and lightly golden. Serve the frittata warm or cold, cut into wedges or strips.

VARIATION
Try adding 1½ cups cooked diced chicken or four slices cooked bacon instead of the tuna. Cooked, sliced link sausages (about four) or 7 oz diced smoked ham could also be used in place of the tuna.

8 months

FLOUNDER WITH ROASTED TOMATOES

If serving to babies as a puree, peel off the skin from the fish after cooking and flake, being careful to remove any bones before combining with the roasted tomatoes and a little water or milk. You could use any type of fish in this recipe.

1 Preheat the oven to 400°F. Heat 1 tablespoon of the oil in a roasting pan and add the tomatoes and basil. Turn the tomatoes in the oil and season with black pepper, if using. Roast for 6–10 minutes, until tender. Peel off the tomato skins.

2 Dust the fish in seasoned flour. Heat half of the butter and a little of the remaining oil in a skillet until hot. Cook two fillets for 4–5 minutes, turning halfway. Keep warm while you cook the remaining flounder.

3 Place the fish on serving plates with the tomatoes and squeeze the lemon juice over the top, if using.

**4 servings
(2 children, 2 adults)**

potato wedges and peas

INGREDIENTS

1½ tablespoons olive oil, plus extra for frying
20 cherry tomatoes
Handful fresh basil
4 flounder fillets
Flour, for dusting
1¾ tablespoons unsalted butter
2 teaspoons lemon juice (optional)

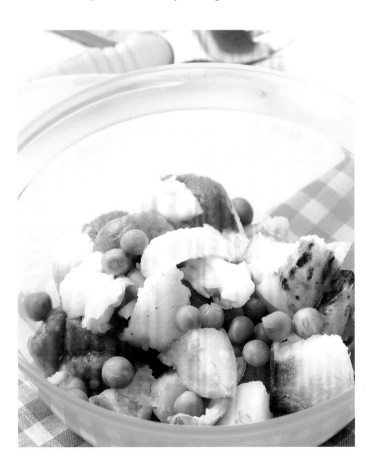

CREAMY FISH CASSEROLE

Perfect comfort food, this complete meal provides a good balance of nutrients, such as low-fat protein, vitamin C, the B vitamins, zinc, and calcium. It's also a great meal for children, but make sure there are no bones in the dish. For babies under 12 months, omit the shrimp.

**4 servings
(2 children, 2 adults)**

**steamed broccoli or
green beans**

INGREDIENTS

2 tablespoons vegetable oil
1 small leek, sliced
   or 1 onion, chopped
1 stick celery, chopped
1 carrot, chopped
1 bay leaf
6 Yukon gold or russet
   potatoes, peeled and halved
   or quartered, if large
2 tablespoons butter, plus
   extra for topping
2 tablespoons all-purpose
   flour
1¼ cups milk
1 teaspoon Dijon mustard
2 tablespoons crème fraîche
8 oz undyed smoked haddock
   fillet or similar smoked fish,
   skinned and cut into
   1-inch pieces
8 oz halibut fillet or similar
   firm white fish, skinned and
   cut into 1-inch pieces
4 oz cooked shrimp, defrosted
   if frozen (optional)
⅔ cup frozen peas

12 months

1   Heat the oil in a large saucepan and sauté the leek, celery, and carrot for 10 minutes, until softened. Add the bay leaf while the vegetables are cooking.

2   Meanwhile, cook the potatoes in plenty of boiling water until tender, and then drain well. Preheat the oven to 350°F.

3   Mash the potatoes with the butter until smooth—you want a dry mashed consistency. Cover the pan with a lid to keep the mashed potatoes warm and set aside.

4   Stir the flour into the softened onions and cook for 1 minute, then gradually add the milk, stirring continuously. When the sauce has thickened, stir in the mustard and crème fraîche and heat through.

5   Add the fish, shrimp, and peas to the white sauce and stir until combined, then spoon the mixture into an ovenproof dish.

6   Top the fish mixture with the mashed potatoes in an even layer. Dot the top with little pats of butter, then bake for about 25 minutes, until golden.

STORAGE TIP
Creamy Fish Casserole (without shrimp) will keep stored in the refrigerator in an airtight container for up to three days or can be frozen for up to three months.

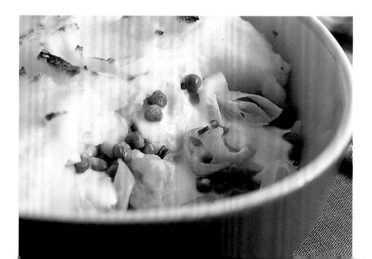

SALMON STICKS WITH SWEET POTATO FRIES

This healthy version of the children's classic fish sticks and french fries offers plenty of brain-boosting omega-3 fatty acids. Children need essential fatty acids provided by the salmon for their rapidly developing brains and nerves. If your baby is unable to handle the sticks, mash or cut into smaller pieces as appropriate.

1 Preheat the oven to 400°F. To make the fries, dry the sweet potatoes on a clean dish towel. Spoon the oil into a roasting pan and heat briefly. Toss the sweet potatoes in the warm oil until covered and roast for 30 minutes, turning them half-way through, until tender and golden.

2 Meanwhile, mix together the cornmeal with the Parmesan on a plate. Dip each salmon stick into the beaten egg, then roll them in the cornmeal-and-Parmesan mixture until evenly coated.

3 Heat enough oil to cover the bottom of a large heavy skillet. Carefully arrange the salmon sticks in the pan and cook them for 6 minutes, turning halfway through, until golden. Drain on kitchen paper then serve with the sweet potato fries.

VARIATION

Try using thick fillets of white fish such as cod, halibut, or Alaskan pollack in place of the salmon.

**4 servings
(2 children, 2 adults)**

peas and carrots

INGREDIENTS

⅔ cup cornmeal or 1 cup dry bread crumbs
3 tablespoons freshly grated Parmesan
12 oz salmon fillet, skinned and sliced into 10 chunky sticks
2 eggs, beaten
sunflower oil, for frying
Black pepper, to taste (optional)

Sweet potato fries
3 sweet potatoes, peeled and cut into wedges
2 tablespoons olive oil

8 months

SALMON FRITTATA

It is recommended that children have at least two portions of fish a week, one of which should be an oily variety, such as salmon. Frittata is a versatile dish and makes a nutritious lunch or supper. Alternatively, cut into wedges and serve as a snack to be eaten with fingers.

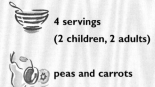

4 servings
(2 children, 2 adults)

peas and carrots

INGREDIENTS

3 white round or red-skinned
   potatoes, peeled and halved
1½ tablespoons olive oil
2 onions, sliced
1 (14¾-oz) can salmon, skin
   and large bones removed
   and fish flaked
2 tablespoons chopped fresh
   parsley (optional)
6 eggs, lightly beaten
Freshly ground black pepper
   (optional)
2 tablespoons unsalted butter

1 Cook the potatoes in plenty of boiling water until tender. Drain the potatoes and set aside.

2 Meanwhile, heat the oil in a large, heavy skillet with an ovenproof handle. Sauté the onions over low heat for 10 minutes, or until softened.

3 Slice the potatoes into disks and put into a large mixing bowl with the salmon, onions, parsley, if using, and eggs. Stir the mixture gently until combined, then carefully pour it into the skillet. Season with black pepper, if using.

4 Preheat the broiler to medium. Cook the frittata over medium-low heat on the stove for about 3 minutes, until the bottom has set and is slightly golden.

5 Place the pan under the preheated broiler for about 2 minutes, until the frittata is slightly golden and set.

VARIATION
Try using canned tuna in spring water, drained, in place of the salmon.

STORAGE TIP
Salmon Frittata will keep stored in the refrigerator for up to two days.

12
months

VEGETABLE SOUP WITH CHICKEN DUMPLINGS

Some children like to be able to identify what they are eating, so they are happy to try pieces of vegetables, while others are more likely to eat up if the dish is pureed; this soup can be served either way. For babies of six months, puree the dumplings with the soup.

1 To make the chicken dumplings, put the chicken, Parmesan, oil, and bread crumbs into a food processor or blender and process to a coarse paste. Season with black pepper, if using, and form into 12 walnut-size balls. Put the balls onto a plate and chill, covered, for 30 minutes, until firm.

2 Heat the oil in a large saucepan and sauté the onion for 5 minutes, stirring frequently, until softened. Next, add the celery, carrots, potatoes, and bay leaves and sauté for another 2 minutes.

3 Pour in the water and add the bouquet garni, then bring to a boil. Reduce the heat and simmer the soup, half-covered, for 10 minutes.

4 Add the chicken balls and cook them for 5–8 minutes, turning them occasionally, until they are cooked through and the soup has reduced slightly.

5 Remove the chicken dumplings with a slotted spoon and set aside. Stir the crème fraîche into the soup and heat through gently. Puree the soup in a blender, if preferred, then season to taste with black pepper, if using.

5 Ladle the soup into four bowls, then distribute the dumplings as appropriate, grinding or chopping them, if necessary.

STORAGE TIP

The Vegetable Soup will keep stored in the refrigerator in an airtight container for up to five days or can be frozen for up to three months. The cooked dumplings can be kept in the refrigerator for up to two days or frozen for up to three months.

**4 servings
(2 children, 2 adults)**

bread

INGREDIENTS

1 tablespoon olive oil
1 large onion, chopped
1 stick celery, diced
2 large carrots, scrubbed
   and diced
2 large Yukon gold or white
   round potatoes, peeled
   and diced
2 bay leaves
5¼ cups water
1 bouquet garni (sprigs of
   parsley, thyme, and bay leaf
   tied together)
2 tablespoons crème fraîche
   (optional)
Freshly ground black pepper
   (optional)

Chicken dumplings
10 oz skinless chicken breasts,
   cubed
¼ cup finely grated Parmesan
   cheese
1½ tablespoons olive oil
⅓ cup fresh bread crumbs
Freshly ground black
   pepper (optional)

BARBECUE CHICKEN WITH COLESLAW

It's a good idea to familiarize children with new and stronger flavors when young, so they will be less likely to become fussy eaters later in life. This barbecue marinade gives the chicken a wonderful color and sweet-sour taste.

 **4 servings
(2 children, 2 adults)**

in place of the coleslaw, you could serve the chicken with steamed broccoli, carrots, and new potatoes

INGREDIENTS

4 skinless, boneless chicken
  breasts

Marinade

3 tablespoons ketchup
2 tablespoons soy sauce
2 tablespoons balsamic or
  sherry vinegar
2 tablespoons maple syrup

Coleslaw

2 tablespoons shredded carrot
2 tablespoons shredded
  green cabbage
1 teaspoon mayonnaise
2 teaspoons plain yogurt
squeeze of lemon juice
1 teaspoon olive oil

1 Mix together the ketchup, soy sauce, vinegar, and maple syrup in a shallow dish. Add the chicken and turn until the breasts are coated in the barbecue sauce. Marinate the chicken for 30 minutes, or longer if you have time, turning the meat occasionally.

2 Meanwhile, preheat the broiler to medium-high and line the broiler pan with aluminum foil.

3 Broil the chicken for about 20 minutes, turning once and spooning more marinade over them, until cooked through. Discard any leftover marinade.

4 While the chicken is cooking, prepare the coleslaw. Put the shredded carrots and cabbage into a bowl. Mix in the mayonnaise, yogurt, lemon juice, and olive oil, then stir until everything is mixed together.

5 Remove the cooked chicken from the broiler and let cool slightly. Cut the chicken into pieces if your baby is able to handle finger foods or if he or she is not ready, grind or finely chop the chicken. Accompany with the coleslaw.

STORAGE TIP

The cooked chicken will keep chilled for up to two days. Store the coleslaw in an airtight container for up to three days.

8-9
months

CHICKEN STICKS

Chicken is an excellent source of low-fat protein, but try to buy organic, free-range meat, if possible. Remove the skewers before serving to babies. If your baby is unable to handle finger foods, puree, grind, or finely chop, depending on his or her age.

1 Soak 16 wooden skewers in a bowl of water for 30 minutes to prevent them from burning. Cut each chicken breast lengthwise into four strips and thread each one onto a skewer.

2 Combine the olive oil, lemon juice, and black pepper, if using, in a small bowl, then brush the chicken with the mixture.

3 Heat a ridged grill pan or broiler to medium-hot. Cook the chicken skewers for 3 minutes on each side, until golden and cooked through, making sure there is no trace of pink inside. Cook for slightly longer if there is any sign of pink.

**4 servings
(2 children, 2 adults)**

**couscous or rice and
corn kernels**

INGREDIENTS

4 skinless, boneless chicken
  breasts
2 tablespoons olive oil
juice of ½ lemon
Black pepper, to taste
  (optional)

6-7
months

ROASTED RED PESTO CHICKEN

Serve this flavorsome roasted chicken with potatoes and plenty of vegetables for
a delicious weekend meal.

**4 servings
(2 children, 2 adults)**

**roasted potatoes
or mashed and**
steamed vegetables

INGREDIENTS

4 skinless, boneless chicken
  breasts
1 tablespoon olive oil
2 tablespoons pine nuts
  (optional)

Red pesto
1 cup drained and chopped
  semi-dried tomatoes in oil
  (or 1 cup sun-dried
  tomatoes in oil soaked in
  water for 2 hours, drained,
  and chopped)
2 garlic cloves, crushed
¼ cup pine nuts
⅔ cup extra-virgin olive oil
½ cup freshly grated
  Parmesan cheese

1 Preheat the oven to 400°F. To make the red pesto, put the
ingredients into a food processor and blend until it forms
a coarse puree.

2 Arrange the chicken in a large ovenproof dish. Brush each
breast with the oil, then spread a tablespoon of red pesto
over each one until completely covered. Roast the chicken for
30 minutes or until the juices run clear when it is pierced with
a the tip of a sharp knife and there is no sign of any pink.

4 Meanwhile, lightly toast the pine nuts in a dry skillet. To serve
as finger food, cut the chicken into pieces, but if your baby is
not ready for finger food, grind or finely chop the chicken. For
older children and adults, arrange the chicken breasts on plates,
sprinkle with the nuts, and serve.

STORAGE TIP

Any leftover pesto can be stored in an airtight container in the
refrigerator for up to a week.

*Note Pesto contains pine nuts—avoid serving to babies if there
is a history of nut allergy, asthma, hay fever, or eczema within the
immediate family. Please consult your pediatrician.*

8
months

CHICKEN BALLS IN TOMATO SAUCE

A great Italian-inspired dish that's popular with kids.

1 To make the balls, mix together the chicken, Parmesan, bread crumbs, and egg. Season with black pepper, if using, and, using floured hands, form into 20 small balls—don't worry about making them perfectly round, because the mixture is moist.

2 Heat enough oil to just cover the bottom of a heavy skillet and cook the balls, in batches if necessary, for 6–8 minutes, turning occasionally, until browned and cooked though. Remove from the pan and keep warm.

3 To make the sauce, heat the olive oil in a saucepan and add the garlic and oregano. Sauté for 30 seconds, then add the diced tomatoes and tomato paste. Cook for 4 minutes over a medium-low heat, stirring occasionally.

4 Return the chicken balls to the pan and cook for another 4 minutes, until heated through and the sauce has reduced and thickened.

5 For babies, puree the chicken balls in the tomato sauce or grind or finely chop, depending on your child's age.

VARIATION
Try using the same quantity of lean ground round beef instead of the chicken to make the balls.

4 servings
(2 children, 2 adults)

pasta or rice and a
green vegetable or
salad

INGREDIENTS

12 oz ground chicken
3 tablespoons freshly grated
  Parmesan cheese
1 cup fresh bread crumbs
1 medium egg, beaten
Black pepper, to taste
  (optional)
Flour, for dusting
Olive oil, for frying

Tomato sauce
1 tablespoon olive oil
1 large garlic clove, crushed
1 teaspoon dried oregano
1 (14½-oz) can diced
  tomatoes
1 tablespoon tomato paste

6
months

TURKEY PATTIES WITH PINEAPPLE RELISH

These patties are made with low-fat turkey and little else. Turkey provides useful amounts of protein and the B vitamins and is generally lower in fat than red meat. The patty comes with a vitamin C-rich pineapple and mint relish.

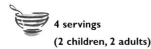

**4 servings
(2 children, 2 adults)**

vegetable sticks

INGREDIENTS

12 oz lean ground turkey
1 teaspoon dried oregano
1 large garlic clove, crushed
  (optional)
Freshly ground black pepper,
  to taste (optional)
Olive oil, for brushing
Burger buns or rolls, to serve;
  use mini rolls for children

Pineapple relish
2 tablespoons finely diced
  canned or fresh peeled
  pineapple
1 tablespoon finely finely
  chopped fresh mint
  (optional)
1½-inch piece cucumber,
  peeled, seeded, and
  finely diced
2 teaspoons lemon juice

1 Mix together the ground turkey, oregano, and garlic, if using, in a mixing bowl. Season with black pepper, if using, and divide the mixture into portions. Use your hands to roll each portion into a ball, then flatten into a patty shape. Put the patties on a plate, cover with plastic wrap, and chill for 30 minutes.

2 Preheat the broiler to medium-high and line the broiler pan with aluminum foil. Meanwhile, mix together the ingredients for the relish and set aside to let the flavors mingle.

3 Brush the patties with oil, then broil them for 3–5 minutes on each side, or until cooked through and there is no trace of pink in the center.

4 To serve, cut the buns in half crosswise and put a patty on top. Add a spoonful of the relish. Top with the second half of the bun.

SERVING TIP
If your baby can manage finger food, cut the patty into pieces and the bun into strips and serve alongside. If your baby isn't ready for finger foods, puree, mash, or grind together the patty and relish.

STORAGE TIP
The patties can be frozen, uncooked, for up to three months. Separate the patties with a small sheet of wax paper to prevent them from sticking together.

8 months

TURKEY FRICASSEE

This is a satisfying and healthy combination of turkey, vegetables, and beans.

1 Sprinkle the flour on a plate and season with black pepper, if using. Toss the turkey pieces in the flour.

2 Heat the oil in a large, heavy lidded sauté pan over medium heat and sauté the onion for 7 minutes. Remove the onion and add the turkey pieces. Cook for 10 minutes, turning the turkey occasionally, until browned all over. (You may need to do this in two batches, adding a little extra oil, if necessary.) Set the turkey aside while you cook the vegetables.

3 Return the onion to the pan and add the garlic, black pepper, oregano, carrots, and corn kernels, then cook for 3 minutes, or until the vegetables have softened. Return the turkey to the pan.

4 Add the water and bring to a boil, then reduce the heat and simmer, covered, for 15 minutes, stirring occasionally. Add the crème fraîche or yogurt and beans and warm through, stirring, for a few minutes before serving. Puree, mash, or grind, if necessary.

STORAGE TIP
The fricassee can be frozen in portions, if desired, for future use. It will keep for up to three months in the freezer. Alternatively, store in the refrigerator in an airtight container for up to two days.

4 servings
(2 children, 2 adults)

rice or mashed
potatoes

INGREDIENTS

1 tablespoon all-purpose flour
Black pepper to taste
  (optional)
1 lb skinless turkey breasts,
  cut into bite-size pieces
1 tablespoon olive oil
1 large onion, finely chopped
2 garlic cloves, chopped
1 red bell pepper, seeded and
  diced
2 teaspoons dried oregano
2 carrots, finely diced
2 corn-on-the-cobs, kernels
  sliced off
1 cup water
¼ cup crème fraîche or plain
  Greek yogurt
1¼ cups drained and rinsed,
  canned cranberry beans or
  pinto beans

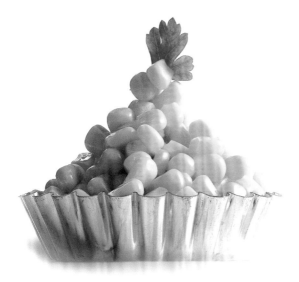

8
months

MEATY PAELLA

Paella rice is perfect for young children, because it has a soft, melt-in-the-mouth texture. The rice is colored with a pinch of saffron, but you could use turmeric instead.

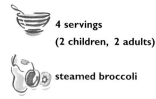

4 servings
(2 children, 2 adults)

steamed broccoli

INGREDIENTS

2 tablespoons olive oil

1 onion, diced

1 red bell pepper, cored, seeded, and diced

2 cloves garlic, finely chopped

2 tomatoes, seeded and diced

Pinch of saffron

2¾ cups hot water

1 cup paella rice or other medium-grain rice

½ cup frozen peas

3 frankfurters, cooked and sliced or finely chopped

1 | Heat the oil in a large skillet. Add the onion and sauté for 8 minutes, or until softened. Add the bell pepper and garlic and cook for another 2 minutes over medium heat.

2 | Add the tomatoes, saffron, and water to the pan. Stir in the rice and bring to a boil, stirring frequently. Reduce the heat and simmer for 20 minutes, stirring occasionally, until the rice is tender and the water has been absorbed.

3 | Stir in the peas and cooked frankfurters and cook for 2 minutes, or until heated through.

VARIATION
Try adding 2 cups cooked diced chicken or ham instead of the frankfurters.

STORAGE TIP
Store Meaty Paella in the refrigerator for up to two days or freeze for up to three months. Reheat until piping hot throughout.

8 months

ROASTED SAUSAGES & POTATOES

There is something comforting about a roast dinner. This weekday version doesn't skimp on the comfort element, but it is a more simple to prepare and cook.

1 Preheat the oven to 400°F. Put the oil into a large roasting pan with the potatoes. Turn the potatoes in the oil and roast in the oven for 10 minutes.

2 Add the sausages, squash, and herbs, stir everything together, and return to the oven for 15 minutes. Combine the hot water and cornstarch in a small bowl and pour the liquid over the sausage mixture.

3 Cook for another 10 minutes, until the liquid has thickened and formed a gravy and the sausages and vegetables are cooked and golden. Remove the herbs and serve.

VARIATION

For a vegetarian version, use nonmeat sausages or alternatively increase the quantity of vegetables. You could use onion, parsnip, celeriac, rutabaga, or beets.

4 servings
(2 children, 2 adults)

green vegetables

INGREDIENTS

2 tablespoons olive oil
8 good-quality link pork
   sausages or vegetarian
   alternative
4 russet potatoes, cut into
   chunks
½ small butternut squash,
   peeled, seeded, and cut into
   chunks the same size as
   the potatoes
2 sprigs fresh rosemary
2 sprigs fresh oregano
10 cherry tomatoes
⅔ cup low-sodium stock
1 tablespoon cornstarch
Black pepper, to taste
   (optional)

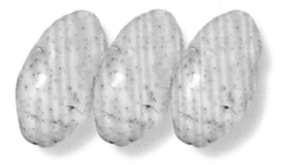

12 months

HAM & PEA PENNE

Try to buy good-quality ham to give the best flavor to this quick and simple pasta dish.
Ham can be salty, so look for reduced-sodium versions if serving this dish to young babies or
only serve it in small quantities.

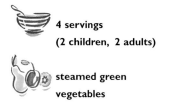

**4 servings
(2 children, 2 adults)**

**steamed green
vegetables**

INGREDIENTS

12 oz penne
1 tablespoon olive oil
2 large cloves garlic, chopped
1 cup water
1 cup frozen peas
½ cup creme fraîche or
   plain Greek yogurt
4 thick slices of cured ham,
   cut into bite-size pieces
Black pepper, to taste
   (optional)
Freshly grated Parmesan
   cheese, to serve

1 Cook the pasta in plenty of boiling water, following the package directions. Drain, reserving 2 tablespoons of the cooking water.

2 Meanwhile, heat the olive oil in a large, heavy skillet and sauté the garlic for 30 seconds. Add the water, followed by the peas, and cook over medium-high heat for 2 minutes, until the peas are cooked and the liquid has reduced.

3 Add the ham to the pan with the creme fraîche. Cook over low heat, stirring frequently, until warmed through. Stir in the pasta and the reserved cooking water, if required, and stir gently until combined. Season with black pepper, if using, and serve sprinkled with Parmesan. Puree, adding a little milk, if serving to babies.

VARIATION
Replace the ham with 5 oz canned tuna or salmon. You could also use fresh cooked salmon, flaked into pieces, or 1 cup cooked, diced chicken.

PORK WITH FRUITY COUSCOUS

The marinade gives the pork a wonderful sweet, glossy glaze. A certain amount
of forward planning is required, because they need to marinate for at least an hour, or you
can let the marinate overnight to absorb the flavors.

1 Mix together the ingredients for the marinade in a shallow, nonmetallic dish. Add the pork and turn until they coated in the marinade. Let marinate in the refrigerator for 1 hour, turning the pork occasionally.

2 To make the couscous, put the couscous in a heatproof bowl. Pour over enough boiling water until it is ¼ inch above the couscous; let the couscous stand until it has absorbed all of the liquid. Add a small pat of butter and fluff up with a fork. Stir in the diced nectarine and set aside.

3 Preheat the broiler to high and line the broiler pan with aluminum foil. Broil the pork for 10–15 minutes, turning halfway and brushing with the marinade, until cooked.

4 Serve the pork with the fruity couscous. Cut the pork into pieces or grind or coarsely chop for babies.

VARIATION
The marinade also works well with poultry, tofu, and salmon.

4 servings
(2 children, 2 adults)

steamed green beans

INGREDIENTS

4 lean pork cutlets

Marinade
2 tablespoons honey
2 tablespoons soy sauce
1 tablespoon balsamic vinegar
1 tablespoon toasted
   sesame oil
2 teaspoons olive oil

Fruity couscous
½ cup couscous
Small pat of butter
1 nectarine or peach, diced
2 tablespoons toasted
   sesame seeds
2 tablespoons toasted
   slivered almonds

12
months

PORK & APPLE PAN-FRY

Pork tenderloin is used here because it is lean and cooks quickly. The apple is perfect with pork and the beans add healthy low-fat protein and minerals.

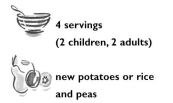

4 servings
(2 children, 2 adults)

new potatoes or rice
and peas

INGREDIENTS

1 tablespoon all-purpose flour
1 teaspoon paprika
1 lb pork tenderloin, trimmed
   and cut into bite-size pieces
1½ tablespoons olive oil
1 large onion, finely chopped
1 large sweet, crisp apple,
   cored, peeled, and cut into
   bite-size pieces
1 tablespoon chopped fresh
   rosemary
1¼ cups water
2 tomatoes, seeded and
   coarsely chopped
1 (15-oz) can cranberry beans
   or pinto beans, drained
   and rinsed
2 tablespoons crème fraîche
   or plain Greek yogurt
Black pepper, to taste
   (optional)

1 Mix together the flour and paprika in a small plastic food bag and add the pork pieces. Shake the bag to toss the pork in the seasoned flour. Turn out the pork onto a plate, shaking off any excess flour. Alternatively, place the flour and paprika on a plate and roll the pork pieces into them to coat.

2 Heat the oil in a heavy skillet, add the pork, and cook for 5 minutes, turning the meat, until browned all over. Add the onion and cook for another 7 minutes, until softened. Mix in the apple and rosemary and cook for 3–4 minutes, until the apples begin to break down.

3 Pour in the water, bring to a boil, then reduce the heat and simmer for 15 minutes, until reduced and thickened. Stir in the tomatoes and beans then cook for another 10 minutes over low heat. Stir in the crème fraîche and heat through before serving. Season with black pepper, if using.

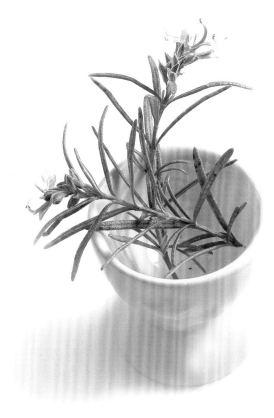

8 months

SPICY GROUND BEEF WITH APRICOTS

This mildly spicy dish can be made in advance and then reheated when ready to serve. The spices can be omitted if preferred, and swapped with 2 teaspoons dried mixed herbs.

1 Heat the oil in a large heavy saucepan, add the onion, and cook, covered, stirring occasionally, over medium heat for 7 minutes, until softened and tender. Add the garlic, carrot, red bell pepper and cook, covered, for another 3 minutes.

2 Push the contents of the pan to one side, add the ground beef, and cook, uncovered, stirring frequently until browned. Stir in the spices and cook for another minute.

3 Pour in the tomato puree and water or broth, then stir in the tomato paste and apricots. Cook, half-covered, for 30-40 minutes, until reduced and thickened. If the sauce appears too liquid, remove the lid; if is it too dry, add a little more water or broth. Season with black pepper, if using, and serve spooned over a baked potato.

VARIATION

You can use a vegetarian alternative instead of the meat or the dish could be used as a base for a casserole. Put the cooked meat (you could omit the apricots) in an ovenproof dish and top with mashed potatoes and shredded cheddar cheese. Cook in an oven, preheated to 400°F, for 25 minutes, until golden on top.

STORAGE TIP

Store in the refrigerator for up to two days or freeze in portions for up to three months.

**4 servings
(2 children, 2 adults)**

**baked potato and
green vegetables**

INGREDIENTS

2 tablespoons olive oil
1 onion, finely chopped
2 cloves garlic, chopped
1 carrot, grated
1 red bell pepper, seeded and diced
1 lb lean ground round beef
½ teaspoon ground cumin
½ teaspoon ground cinnamon
½ teaspoon ground coriander
2 cups tomato puree or tomato sauce
1 cup water or low-sodium vegetable broth
1 tablespoon tomato paste
10 unsulphured dried apricots, finely chopped
Black pepper, to taste (optional)

8 months

MEAT BALLS WITH TOMATO SAUCE

Meat balls accompanied by a smooth tomato sauce are great served with vegetables or over a dish of pasta.

**4 servings
(2 children, 2 adults)**

pasta or steamed
green vegetables, such
as broccoli

INGREDIENTS

Meat balls
12 oz lean ground round beef
1 onion, grated
1 carrot, finely grated
1 clove garlic, crushed
1 cup fresh whole-wheat
  bread crumbs
1 medium egg, beaten
1 tablespoon all-purpose flour
Vegetable oil, for frying

Tomato sauce
1 carrot, finely chopped
1 tablespoon olive oil, plus
  extra for frying
1 clove garlic, crushed
1 (14½-oz) can diced
  tomatoes
1 tablespoon tomato paste

1 Combine the beef, onion, carrot, garlic, bread crumbs, egg, and flour in a bowl. Season to taste and place in the refrigerator for about 1 hour, until the mixture is firm.

2 To make the tomato sauce, blanch the carrots in boiling water for 2–3 minutes, until softened. Heat the oil in a heavy saucepan and sauté the garlic for 1 minute. Add the tomatoes and tomato paste, then cook for 15 minutes, until reduced and thickened. Add the carrots and heat through. Transfer to a blender or food processor and puree until smooth.

3 Form the meat mixture into walnut-size balls, using floured hands. Heat enough oil to cover the bottom of a heavy skillet. Cook the balls, in batches, for about 10 minutes, turning occasionally, until browned all over and cooked.

4 Reheat the tomato sauce, if necessary, and spoon into bowls. Top with the balls and serve. If necessary, cut the balls into pieces or coarsely chop or puree in the tomato sauce.

8 months

HOMEMADE HAMBURGERS

By using good-quality, preferably organic, ingredients, you can have a healthy and delicious hamburger in next to no time. If your baby cannot manage finger food, serve the patty (without the bun) mashed, ground, or cut up.

1 Put the oregano, onion, carrot, garlic, beef, and egg into a large bowl. Season with the black pepper, if using, and mix with your hands until all the ingredients are combined.

2 Divide the mixture into portions and then, using floured hands, form each portion into a patty shape. Set aside in the refrigerator for 15 minutes.

3 Heat enough oil to lightly cover the bottom of a large, heavy skillet. Place the patties in the hot oil and cooked for about 5 minutes on each side, until browned and cooked through.

4 Serve the burgers in buns with relish and accompaniments of choice or cut up into pieces.

**4 servings
(2 children, 2 adults)**

sliced tomato and cucumber; relish, mayonnaise, or ketchup; or boiled potatoes and steamed vegetables

INGREDIENTS

1 teaspoon dried oregano
1 onion, grated
1 carrot, finely grated
1 garlic clove, crushed
1 lb ground chuck beef
1 medium egg, beaten
Black pepper, to taste
   (optional)
Flour, for dusting
Sunflower oil, for frying
Burger buns or rolls, to serve

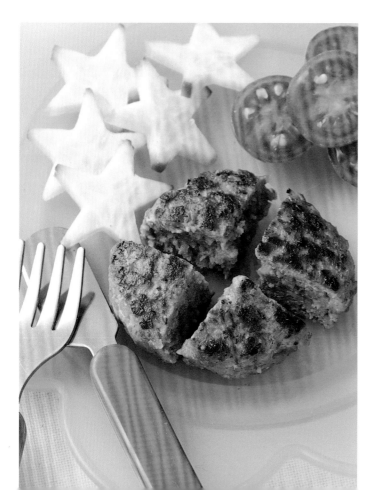

8 months

HEARTY BEEF STEW

It is important to use the good-quality organic beef for this hearty stew. Don't be put off by the length of time it takes to cook, because it doesn't require any lengthy involvement from the cook and the slow-cooking results is a rich, thick gravy and succulent meat.

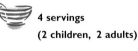

4 servings
(2 children, 2 adults)

mashed potatoes and
a green vegetable

INGREDIENTS

3 tablespoons flour
1 lb boneless beef chuck
   or beef round, diced
3 tablespoons olive oil
8–10 shallots, peeled and
   halved or quartered, if large
2 carrots, cut into batons
1 parsnip, sliced into disks
2 bay leaves
1 tablespoon chopped
   fresh rosemary
1 tablespoon chopped
   fresh thyme
2 cups water
1 cup apple juice
1 tablespoon Worcestershire
   sauce
18 drained canned chestnuts
Black pepper, to taste
   (optional)

1 Preheat the oven to 325°F. Put the flour into a clean plastic food bag or on a plate. Toss the beef in the flour until coated. Heat 1 tablespoon of the oil in a large casserole dish.

2 Add one-third of the beef and cook for 5–6 minutes, turning occasionally, until browned all over—the meat may stick to the pan until it is properly sealed. Remove the browned beef from the pan and cook the remaining two batches, adding another 1 tablespoon oil when necessary. Set aside when all the beef has been browned.

3 Add the remaining oil to the pan with the shallots, carrots, parsnip, and herbs and cook for 3 minutes, stirring occasionally.

4 Pour in the water and bring to a boil. Cook over high heat until the liquid has reduced. Add the apple juice and Worcestershire sauce, then cook for another 3 minutes.

5 Stir in the chestnuts and beef, cover the casserole dish with a lid, and transfer to the oven. Cook for 2 hours, until the stock has formed a thick, rich gravy and the meat is tender. Season with black pepper, if using, before serving.

STORAGE TIP
Hearty Beef Stew will keep stored in the refrigerator in an airtight container for up to three days or can be frozen for up to three months.

8 months

CHINESE BEEF WITH NOODLES

Beef is a good source of iron, although chicken or pork and vegetables of your choice can be used to make this speedy dinner dish, if preferred. Coarsely puree, ground, or finely chop all the ingredients, depending on the age of your baby.

1 Heat the oil in a wok or large, heavy skillet and add the beef, then stir-fry over medium-high heat for 2 minutes. Remove the beef, using a slotted spoon, and set aside.

2 Meanwhile, bring a large saucepan of water to a boil. Add the noodles, stirring to separate them, and follow the package directions to prepare them. Drain when the noodles are tender and keep them warm.

3 Add the garlic, sugar snap peas, and scallions to the wok and stir-fry for 2 minutes, then return the beef to the wok with the black bean and soy sauces; stir-fry for another minute, adding a splash of water if the sauce begins to dry out.

4 Divide the noodles among the plates, then top with the beef stir-fry.

STORAGE TIP
Chinese Beef with Noodles can be stored in an airtight container in the refrigerator for up to two days. Reheat thoroughly before serving.

4 servings
(2 children, 2 adults)

serve with a glass of fresh orange juice to enhance the absorption of the iron in the beef

INGREDIENTS

2 tablespoons sunflower oil
  or vegetable oil
I lb lean beef, cut into strips
8 oz medium egg noodles
3 cloves garlic
2 handfuls sugar snap peas,
  trimmed
I red bell pepper, seeds
  removed and cut into
  ½-inch strips
4 scallions, sliced diagonally
¾ cup black bean sauce
2 tablespoons reduced-
  sodium soy sauce

8-9 months

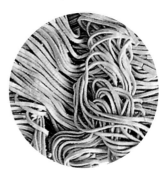

FRUIT YOGURT SWIRLS

Making your own fruit yogurt couldn't be more simple, and it also means you know exactly what's in it. Frozen fruit—either single fruit or mixed—is an excellent alternative to fresh and still counts toward the recommended number of fruits and vegetables you should have daily.

 1–4 child-size servings

INGREDIENTS

¼ cup mixed red berries,
  defrosted if frozen
I nectarine, halved, pitted,
  and quartered
3–4 tablespoons water
plain Greek yogurt, to serve

6 months

1 Put the berries, nectarine, and water into a saucepan with a lid. Bring to simmering point, then cover the pan and cook for 5–7 minutes, until the berries and plums are soft and beginning to break down.

2 Press the cooked fruit through a strainer to remove any seeds and skin.

3 Spoon a serving of yogurt into a glass or bowl. Add a few spoonfuls of the fruit puree and swirl it into the yogurt, using a spoon handle to create a marbled effect.

STORAGE TIP
Any leftover fruit puree can be stored for up to three days in an airtight container in the refrigerator.

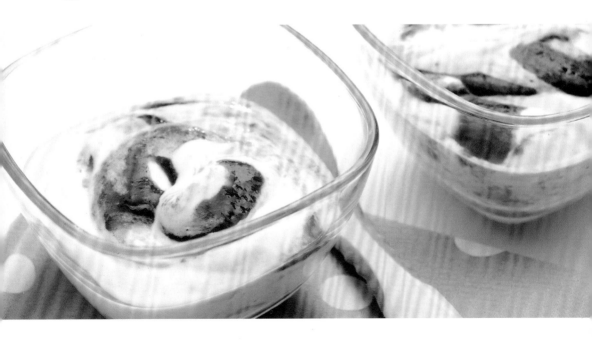

MANGO WHIP

This creamy dessert can be whipped up in a matter of minutes.

1 | Put the mango into a food processor or blender, reserving four slices to decorate. Puree the mango until smooth.

4 servings
(2 children, 2 adults)

2 Add the cream, sugar, and yogurt and blend until combined.

INGREDIENTS

3 Spoon the mixture into dessert glasses and refrigerate for 1 hour, until slightly firm.

1 large mango, pitted, peeled, and coarsely chopped
1 cup heavy cream
2 teaspoons confectioners' sugar or fruit syrup
¼ cup plain yogurt

VARIATION

Any of your favorite fruit can be used instead of the mango, but make sure it has a soft flesh. Apples and pears or other similar fruit with a firmer flesh will first need cooking.

8 months

REAL FRUIT ICE POPS

Homemade ice pops are lower in sugar than most commercially made ones, and they are certainly free from artificial colors and other E numbers.

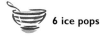 **6 ice pops**

INGREDIENTS

4 plums, halved and pitted
3 nectarines, pitted and
   coarsely chopped
1 tablespoon superfine sugar,
   to taste
⅔ cup prepared custard

6 months

1 Put the plums and nectarines into a medium, nonmetallic saucepan. Add the sugar and 2 tablespoons water. Bring to a boil, then reduce the heat and simmer for 5 minutes, until softened.

2 Let cool, then puree until smooth; you will need about 1 cup.

3 Combine the fruit puree and custard, then spoon the mixture into six ice pop molds. Place in the freezer until solid.

VARIATION
Orange and mango are refreshing alternatives. Juice the fruit—you need about 1¾ cups to make six ice pops—then freeze until solid.

BANANA & MAPLE YOGURT ICE

This simple alternative to ice cream couldn't be easier to make, and it's the perfect dessert for soothing sore gums and for relieving teething pain.

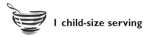 **1 child-size serving**

INGREDIENTS

1 small ripe banana
1 heaping tablespoon
   plain Greek yogurt
1 teaspoon maple syrup
   (optional)

1 Peel the banana, wrap it tightly in plastic film, and freeze for at least 3 hours, until firm—although it can be stored in the freezer until ready to use.

2 Remove the frozen banana from the freezer and unwrap. Let stand for 15 minutes to soften slightly, then break into chunks.

3 Put the banana into a food processor or blender with the yogurt and maple syrup, if using, and blend until thick, smooth, and creamy. Spoon the ice into a bowl.

STORAGE TIP
The Banana & Yogurt Ice will keep stored in the refrigerator in an airtight container for up to two days, but it will defrost after an hour, becoming a fruit whip. The banana can be stored in the freezer for up to three months.

6 months

STRAWBERRY SUNDAE

You can't go wrong with an ice cream sundae. This popular dessert is a breeze to make and has been adapted to ensure a healthy twist.

1 Puree the strawberries and orange juice in a food processor or blender until smooth.

2 Lightly toast the almonds or chopped nuts in a dry skillet. Set aside.

3 To serve, place a few spoonfuls of the strawberry sauce in a tall glass. Top with a scoop of ice cream and another spoonful of sauce. Add a final scoop of ice cream. Sprinkle the nuts over the top and a few shavings of chocolate. Repeat to make another sundae.

Note This recipe contains nuts; avoid serving to babies if there is a history of nut allergy, asthma, hay fever, or eczema within the immediate family. Please consult your pediatrician.

2 child-size servings

INGREDIENTS

1 cup hulled and halved strawberries
1 tablespoon fresh orange juice
1 tablespoon slivered almonds or chopped nuts
4 scoops good-quality vanilla ice cream
chocolate shavings, to serve (optional)

8 months

- -

STRAWBERRY YOGURT ICE

These fruity yogurt ice pops are particularly refreshing on a hot day and are great for teething infants. Honey should not be given to infants under 12 months (see page 9).

1 Put the strawberries and yogurt into a food processor or blender and process until smooth. Stir in the honey.

2 Pour the strawberry mixture into ice pop molds and freeze for 2–3 hours, until solid.

4 ice pops

INGREDIENTS

1 cup hulled strawberries
½ cup plain Greek yogurt
2 tablespoons honey

12 months

QUICK BERRY BREAD PUDDING

This speedy version of the classic summer dessert takes a fraction of the time to prepare. It features pureed fruit for children who dislike seeds and lumps. A heart-shape cookie cutter is used here, but you can use whatever shape you have on hand.

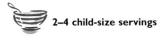 **2–4 child-size servings**

INGREDIENTS

2 cups mixed berries, fresh or
   frozen
⅓ cup fresh apple juice
4 slices day-old white bread,
   crusts removed
Large heart-shape
   cookie cutter

1 Put the berries (reserving a few to decorate) and apple juice into a saucepan and bring to a gentle boil. Reduce the heat and simmer for 5 minutes, until the fruit is soft but there is still plenty of juice.

2 Strain the juice from the fruit through a strainer into a bowl. In a separate bowl, press the fruit through the strainer, using the back of a spoon—this will make a thick puree. Discard any seeds left in the strainer.

3 Cut the bread into heart shapes, using a large cookie cutter—use four slices of bread to make four heart shapes. (The cutter should use as much of each slice as possible, because the bread loses its shape if it is cut too small.)

4 Place two of the hearts in a shallow dish, then spoon over the fruit puree until completely covered. Top the fruit-soaked bread with the remaining two hearts and spoon the juice over them. Press down lightly to soak the juice into the bread. Let stand for 30 minutes. Decorate with the remaining berries to serve.

VARIATION
If preferred, you can omit the bread and combine the cooked pureed berries with plain yogurt.

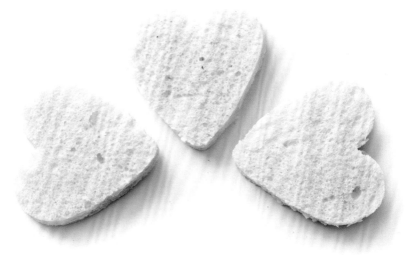

8 months

MIXED FRUIT COMPOTE

Many children dislike "lumps," which can mean they will try to avoid berries. This compote is strained to remove an offending seeds and skin, resulting in an intensely fruity red sauce. You can buy bags of mixed frozen fruit in supermarkets.

1 Put the berries into a saucepan with the apple juice and water, then simmer until defrosted.

2 Add the cornstarch to the pan and heat gently and briefly, stirring frequently, until thickened.

3 Press the fruit through a strainer to remove any seeds.

VARIATION
This fruit compote is delicious stirred into a plain yogurt with a sprinkling of granola.

4–6 child-size servings

INGREDIENTS
2 cups frozen berries, such as
   raspberries, blackberries,
   and hulled and halved or
   quartered strawberries
2 tablespoons apple juice
2 tablespoons water
I teaspoon cornstarch

6 months

APPLE & CINNAMON COMPOTE

This lightly spiced apple compote makes a delicious filling for a warmed croissant. It also can be pureed and stirred into plain yogurt for a healthier version of fruit yogurt.

1 Put the apple, cinnamon, butter, lemon juice (prevents the apple from browning), and water into a heavy, nonmetallic saucepan. Simmer, half-covered, over medium heat for 15 minutes, until the apples are tender.

2 Lightly mash the apples with a fork to break them down slightly or puree in a blender.

VARIATION
Pears would make a delicious alternative to the apple here, as would plums.

STORAGE TIP
Double the quantity of this recipe and freeze in convenient-size portions for future use.

2–4 child-size servings

INGREDIENTS
2 sweet, crips apples, cored,
   peeled, and coarsely diced
½ teaspoon ground cinnamon
small pat of butter
squeeze fresh lemon juice
⅓ cup water

6 months

SNOW BALLS

Packed with energy-giving and iron-boosting dried fruit and nutritious nuts and seeds, these coconut-coated balls make an excellent snack or dessert.

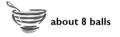 **about 8 balls**

INGREDIENTS

¼ cup coarsely chopped
   hazelnuts
⅓ cup whole oats
⅓ cup raisins
⅔ cup dried unsulfured
   apricots, cut into small pieces
2 tablespoons fresh orange
   juice
1 tablespoon sunflower seeds
1 tablespoon pumpkin seeds
Dried coconut flakes,
   for coating

*Note This recipe contains
nuts; avoid serving to babies
if there is a history of
allergy, asthma, hay fever,
or eczema within the
immediate family. Please
consult your pediatrician.*

1 Put the hazelnuts and oats into a dry skillet and toast over medium heat for 3 minutes, turning them frequently with a wooden spatula until they begin to turn golden and the oats become crisp. Let cool.

2 Put the raisins, apricots, and orange juice into a food processor or blender and puree until the mixture becomes a smooth, thick puree. Scrape the fruit puree into a mixing bowl.

3 Put the nuts, oats, and seeds iton the food processor or blender and process until they are finely chopped. Transfer the mixture to the bowl with the fruit puree. Stir the fruit mixture until all the ingredients are combined.

4 Cover the bowl with plastic wrap and chill the mixture for 1 hour. Scoop up a portion of the fruit-and-nut mixture— about the size of a walnut—in a spoon and roll it into a ball. Rolling is easier if you first form it into a coarse ball, then roll it in the coconut and continue to roll it.

5 Coat the ball in the dried coconut until it is covered, then repeat to make about eight balls in total. Arrange the balls on a plate, cover loosely with plastic wrap, and chill for about 30 minutes, until firm.

STORAGE TIP
Store Snow Balls in an airtight container for up to two weeks.

8-9
months

OAT COOKIES

These favorite cookies are packed with nutritious oats.

1 Preheat the oven to 350°F. Line two baking sheets with parchment paper.

2 Beat together the butter and sugar in a mixing bowl until light and fluffy. Stir in both types of flour, baking powder, and oats, then mix well to make a soft dough.

3 Divide the dough into 12 pieces. Roll each piece into a ball and arrange on the baking sheets, well spaced apart to allow room for the dough to spread. Flatten the top of each ball slightly and bake for 15–20 minutes, until the cookies are just golden but still soft in the center.

4 Let cool 5 minutes, then transfer to wire racks.

12 cookies

INGREDIENTS

1 stick unsalted butter

⅓ cup firmly packed light brown sugar

⅔ cup all-purose flour

3 tablespoons whole wheat flour

¾ teaspoon baking powder

1 cup whole roll oats

12 months

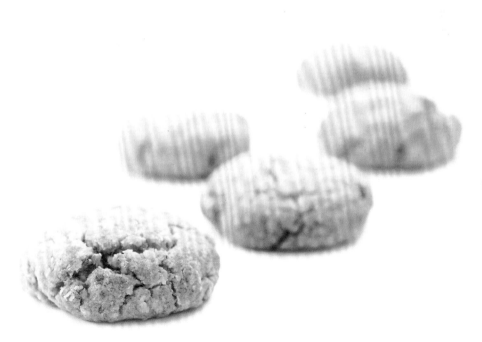

PEACH CRISPS

This variation on the classic crisp uses whole fruits—perfect if you are just cooking for the children, because it's easier to make small portions.

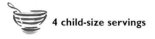 **4 child-size servings**

INGREDIENTS

2 peaches, halved and
   pits removed
3 tablespoons
   all-purpose flour
2 tablespoons unsalted butter
1 tablespoon rolled oats
   (optional)
2 tablespoons raw sugar

8 months

1 Preheat the oven to 350°F. Grease an ovenproof dish or baking pan and arrange the peach halves in the dish.

2 For a crumb topping, put the flour and butter into a bowl and rub together with your fingertips until resembling coarse bread crumbs. Stir in the oats and sugar and mix well.

3 Spoon the crumb mixture over the peaches and add 2 tablespoons of water to the dish. Bake for 25 minutes, or until the peaches are tender and the crumb topping slightly crisp.

VARIATION

Plums, apples, pears, or nectarines make delicious alternatives to the peaches. If you have any leftover crumb mixture, store it in a container or bag in the freezer for future use.

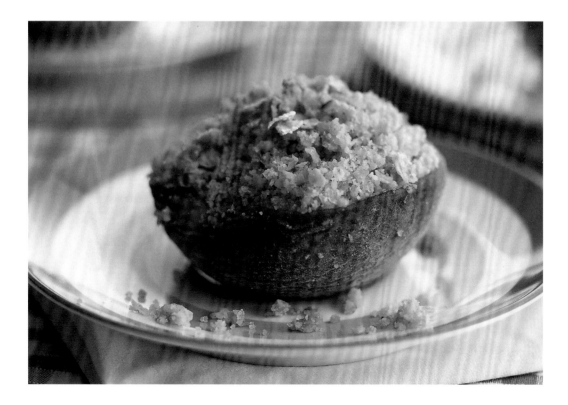

STICKY DATE CAKE

Delicious and light, this makes a great special treat dessert with whipped cream, ice cream, or yogurt or serve on its own for an afternoon snack.

1 Preheat the oven to 350°F. Grease and line the bottom of an 8-inch square cake pan with parchment paper.

2 Put the dates into a medium saucepan with the water. Bring to a boil, then reduce the heat and simmer for about 10 minutes, or until the fruit is soft. Puree the fruit using a handheld blender.

3 Stir the baking soda into the pureed fruit—it will froth up initially—then add the butter.

4 Meanwhile, in a large mixing bowl, whisk the eggs and sugar using an electric handheld mixer for about 8 minutes, until thick and creamy. Gradually sift in the flour and baking powder and gently fold in, using a wooden spoon. Next, fold in the dried fruit mixture and the vanilla.

5 Pour the cake batter into the prepared pan and bake for 35–40 minutes, or until a toothpick inserted in the middle comes out clean. Let stand for 10 minutes, turn out of the pan, and cut into squares.

STORAGE TIP
Store the Sticky Date Cake in an airtight tin or wrapped in aluminum foil for up to one week.

about 16 squares

INGREDIENTS
1½ cups coarsely chopped dried dates
1¼ cups water
1 teaspoon baking soda
4 tablespoons butter, softened, diced
2 extra-large eggs
¾ cup superfine sugar or granulated sugar
1⅓ cups all-purpose flour, sifted
1¼ teaspoons baking powder
1 teaspoon vanilla extract

12 months

CARROT CAKE SQUARES

Your child will never guess that this light and moist cake contains healthy carrots.

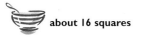 **about 16 squares**

INGREDIENTS

1¾ cups all-purpose flour

1¾ teaspoons baking powder

Pinch of salt

1 teaspoon ground cinnamon

1 teaspoon ground allspice

1 cup firmly packed light
   brown sugar

2 cups peeled and shredded
   carrots

3 large eggs, lightly beaten

¾ cup sunflower oil

1 Preheat the oven to 350°F. Lightly grease an 8-inch square cake pan and line the bottom with wax paper.

2 Sift the flour, baking powder, salt, and spices into a large mixing bowl. Add the sugar and carrots and mix well.

3 Mix together the eggs and oil in a small bowl, then pour into the flour mixture, stirring with a wooden spoon until combined.

4 Pour the cake batter into the prepared cake pan and bake for 50 minutes, or until a toothpick inserted into the center of the cake comes out clean. Let cool for 10 minutes, then carefully turn out the cake and let cool completely before cutting into small squares.

STORAGE TIP
Store the Carrot Cake Squares in an airtight container or wrapped in aluminum foil for up to one week.

LEMON SYRUP CAKES

These individual sponge cakes are baked, unlike the steamed versions they are based on, which drastically cuts down on the cooking time without loosing any flavor.

1 Preheat the oven to 350°F. Grease six dariole molds or ramekins and place on a baking sheet.

2 To make the topping, mix together the corn syrup and lemon juice with a fork.

3 To make the cakes, beat the butter and sugar in a bowl until pale and fluffy. Beat in the eggs, one at a time, beating the mixture thoroughly after each addition—the mixture may curdle but do not worry about this. Beat in the maple syrup.

4 Add half of the flour with the baking powder and fold in with a metal spoon. Add the rest of the flour and fold in.

5 Place a spoonful of the syrup topping into each mold or ramekin, reserving about half of the mixture to serve. Spoon the sponge batter over the topping until it nearly reaches the top and smooth the top with the back of a teaspoon. Bake for 20 minutes or until the cakes are risen and golden.

6 Remove from the oven and let cool for 5 minutes, then run a knife around the edge of the molds or ramekins to loosen the cakes. Heat the remaining syrup mixture until warm. Turn out the cakes onto serving plates and spoon the warm syrup over them.

makes 6

ice cream

INGREDIENTS

Topping
½ cup light corn syrup
2 tablespoons lemon juice

Cakes
1 stick unsalted butter, softened, plus extra for greasing
½ cup firmly packed light brown sugar
3 eggs
1 tablespoon maple syrup
1 cup all-purpose flour
1 teaspoon baking powder

12 months

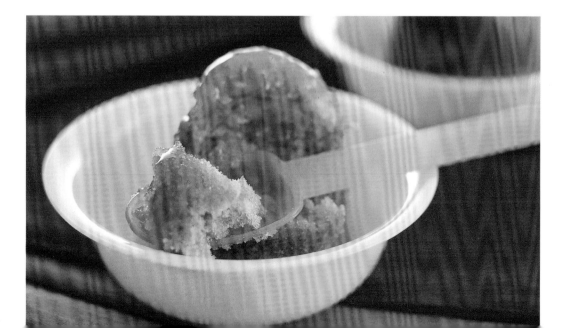

MERRY BERRY COBBLER

Berries are rich in antioxidants and vitamin C. Here, they are used as base for a warming dessert that has a delicious biscuit topping.

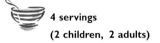 **4 servings**
(2 children, 2 adults)

INGREDIENTS

2 cups mixed berries, such as
   raspberries, blackberries,
   strawberries, blueberries,
   defrosted if frozen
8 plums, halved, pitted, and
   coarsely chopped
1 teaspoon cornstarch
3 tablespoons superfine sugar
   or granulated sugar

Topping
1 stick unsalted butter
2 tablespoons superfine sugar
   or granulated sugar
1⅔ cups all-purpose flour
2 teaspoons baking powder
2 teaspoons cornstarch
1–2 tablespoons light cream

1 Preheat the oven to 350°F. Put the berries and plums into an 8 x 10-inch baking dish. Mix the cornstarch with a little water and add to the fruit with the sugar, stir until thoroughly combined.

2 For the topping, beat the butter and sugar until pale and fluffy. Mix in the flour, baking powder, and cornstarch. As the mixture becomes dry, stir in the cream to form a smooth soft dough.

3 Divide the dough into eight balls, flatten the top of each one, and arrange on top of the berry mixture. Bake for 20–25 minutes, until the biscuit topping is risen and golden.

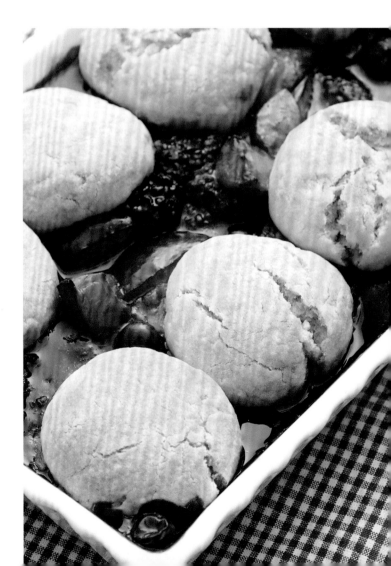

 8-9 months

APPLE, PLUM & OATY CRISP

Fruit crisp with a twist: This dessert has a crisp nutty, oaty topping. You can vary the fruit base according to what's in season—rhubarb, nectarines, berries, and pears are equally delicious. Dessert apples are used here instead of cooking apples, because they don't need as much sugar to sweeten them. Make in individual dishes or one large dish, depending what you have on

1 Preheat the oven to 350°F. Toss the apples in the lemon juice to prevent them from browning and arrange in a 9-inch diameter ovenproof dish with the plums; stir well to combine.

2 To make the topping, melt the syrup and butter in a heavy, medium saucepan. Remove from the heat and stir in the oats, hazelnuts, and seeds. Sprinkle the mixture over the top of the fruit. Bake for 20–25 minutes, until golden and beginning to crisp.

STORAGE TIP
The dessert can be kept in the freezer for up to three months; defrost, then reheat in the oven covered in aluminum foil. Alternatively, freeze the cooked fruit mixture and uncooked crumb topping separately and follow the recipe above for cooking directions.

4-6 servings
(2 children, 2–4 adults)

INGREDIENTS

3 sweet, crisp apples, cored, peeled, and diced
squeeze of lemon juice
5 plums, halved, pitted, and diced

Topping
¼ cup light corn syrup
5 tablespoons unsalted butter
2 cups rolled oats
2 tablespoons chopped hazelnuts
2 tablespoons sunflower seeds

8-9 months

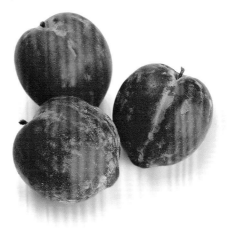

INDEX

INDEX

ACKNOWLEDGMENTS

The publishers would like to thank:

Photographer: Jules Selmes
Photographer's assistant: Adam Giles
Food Stylist: Clare Lewis

For use of images and equipment:
BabyBjörn, www.babybjorn.com
Mothercare, www.mothercare.com